MUSCULOSKELETAL
ASSESSMENT
AN INTEGRATED APPROACH

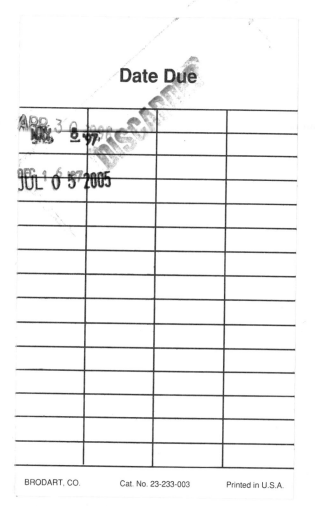

MUSCULOSKELETAL ASSESSMENT
AN INTEGRATED APPROACH

Barbara M. Edwardson, M.Ed.
Department of Physical Therapy
The University of Western Ontario
London, Ontario
Canada

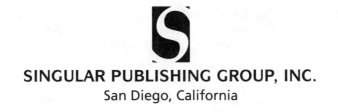

SINGULAR PUBLISHING GROUP, INC.
San Diego, California

Singular Publishing Group, Inc.
4284 41st Street
San Diego, California 92105-1197

Typeset in 10/12 New Century Schoolbook by House Graphics
Printed in the United States of America by McNaughton & Gunn

Library of Congress Cataloging-in-Publication Data
Edwardson, Barbara M., 1929-
    Musculoskeletal assessment: an integrated approach / Barbara M.
Edwardson.
        p.   cm.
    Includes bibliographical references and index.
    ISBN 1-879105-69-1
    1. Musculoskeletal system—Diseases—Diagnosis. 2. Physical
therapy.   I. Title.
    [DNLM: 1. Joint Diseases—diagnosis. 2. Joints—physiology.
3. Movement—physiology. 4. Muscular Diseases—diagnosis.
5. Spinal Injuries—diagnosis. WE 141 E26m]
    RC925.7.E39   1992
    616.7'075—dc20
    DNLM/DLC
    for Library of Congress   92-13349
                                                                    CIP

CONTENTS

To the memory of my parents
and my sister
and
my family of friends

PREFACE

This book has evolved over many years of teaching musculo-skeletal assessment to students at The University of Western Ontario, Canada. Its birth was in the form of course notes; its growth was in the development of manuals; and its maturity is in the completion of this book. *Musculoskeletal Assessment: An Integrated Approach* provides physical therapy students and graduates with the means of assessing patients with musculos-keletal problems utilizing an integrated approach. Not all the available assessment techniques or special tests are contained within these pages. I have utilized an eclectic approach based on common musculoskeletal conditions that exist and the assessment techniques necessary to detect them.

The philosophical approaches in this book are those of the "Masters" of physical therapy, and it is from their writings and teachings that this book has become a reality. I am indebted to the late Dr. James Cyriax for his systematic assessment in orthopedic medicine and his theory of selective tissue tension; to Professor Freddie Kaltenborn for his focus on arthrokinemat-ics in the assessment and treatment of joint problems; to Geoffrey Maitland for his segmental approach to assessment and treatment of the spine; and, finally, to Robin McKenzie for his enlightening contribution to the assessment and treatment of spinal musculoskeletal problems. Readers of this book would benefit enormously from the teachings and writings of these "Masters."

The first three chapters are devoted to the philosophical concepts that are the basis of the assessment process. The remaining nine chapters present detailed examinations of the joints and soft tissue structures that form the dynamic aspect of the musculoskeletal system.

I would like to emphasize the importance of the subjective examination in the assessment procedure. If one **listens to the patient,** the information provided will lead to the cause of the patient's problem. Too often information is ignored, either because it does not fit into the therapist's mind set or because decisions have been made without hearing the patient out. We do not know all there is to know about the musculoskeletal system; perhaps if we listen more to our patients, our knowledge will be improved.

Finally, respect for the patient's dignity and comfort during the objective examination is paramount. We must never lose sight of the fact that the patient is a human being who through adversity, not choice, is seeking our help.

ACKNOWLEDGMENTS

Inevitably in an undertaking of this kind there is a lot of behind the scenes assistance and support. I am indebted to Sally Morgan for her tremendous input and meticulous approach to the editing of this manuscript, to Pat Darling for her calm assurance and encouragement and for incorporating the edited changes into the present manuscript, to Margaret Lee for her secretarial support and personal encouragement with the production of the manuals over the years, to Dr. Daniel Ling without whose encouragement and support this book would forever be in the process of revision, to Jane Lee Ling for the artwork that helped to bring the book to life. Finally, I am indebted to all those students over the years whose questions are responsible for the logistics and comprehensiveness of *Musculoskeletal Assessment: An Integrated Approach.*

CHAPTER 1

• • • • • • • •

Philosophical Approach to Musculoskeletal Assessment

MAJOR CONTRIBUTORS TO PHYSICAL THERAPY

There are many people who have contributed to the process of musculoskeletal assessment. Included in this group are four "Masters": Cyriax, Kaltenborn, Maitland, and McKenzie. Their approaches are utilized by physical therapists to assess and treat muscle and joint problems.

Cyriax

James Cyriax, an English physician, developed a meticulous, systematic approach to the assessment of soft tissue injuries. His approach involves observation, subjective examination (taking the patient's history), objective examination (utilization of movements and special tests to elicit signs and symptoms of injuries), palpation of soft tissue structures, and sensory testing.

Kaltenborn

Freddie Kaltenborn, a Norwegian physiotherapist, with training in chiropracty and osteopathy, utilizes specific translatoric movements of traction and gliding in his approach to examination and treatment.

Maitland

Geoffrey Maitland, an Australian physiotherapist, focuses on eliciting and treating signs and symptoms rather than on specific diagnosis. The change in the patient's signs and symptoms guides the therapist in selecting treatment approaches. Maitland utilizes graded passive movements performed in an oscillatory manner for assessment and treatment. His subjective examination is both detailed and specific, and his objective examination focuses on joints that lie beneath the painful area, joints that refer pain to the painful area, and muscles beneath the painful area.

McKenzie

Robin McKenzie is a New Zealand physical therapist. His area of specialty is the assessment and treatment of back and neck problems, specifically postural problems, derangement, and dysfunction. He uses repeated movements to determine the cause of the patient's problem and selected movements to treat the problem. He is a believer in the "hands off" approach, unless a manual procedure is absolutely necessary, and prefers instead to teach the patient certain exercises to perform on a regular basis. In addition, he educates the patient in the maintenance of good posture under all circumstances.

CONCEPTS OF JOINT MOVEMENT

Passive Movements Used in the Assessment Procedure

There are essentially two types of passive movements, physiological and accessory.

Passive Physiological Movements

These are the movements over which the person has active control and which can also be performed passively, for example, abduction at the glenohumeral joint. The patient can actively abduct the arm through the available range of motion. This is described as the **physiological movement** of the joint. The joint can also be moved passively through the available range of motion and this is called the **passive physiological movement.**

Passive Accessory Movements

These are the movements that occur between two articular surfaces. They are of small amplitude compared with the physiological passive movement and are not under the voluntary control of the patient. They are produced passively and occur in conjunction with a physiological movement to obtain full range of motion. In fact, it is impossible to achieve full range of motion if the accessory movements are restricted. Mennell (1964) describes the accessory movements as "joint play" movements.

All joints exhibit a certain degree of joint play due to looseness of the capsule and ligaments. This is essential for normal function to occur. Tightness of these soft structures results in hypomobility, and lengthening results in hypermobility.

Both the passive physiological movement and the passive accessory movements are tested in the assessment procedure to determine the cause of restriction of joint motion.

Kaltenborn's Translatoric Movements These are passive accessory movements that are divided into traction (or separation) occurring perpendicular to the joint surfaces and gliding (or parallel movement) which takes place parallel to the joint surface. Translatoric movements are used both in assessment and treatment (Kaltenborn, 1989).

Traction There are three grades of traction.

- Traction I: This is almost imperceptible and is sufficient only to eliminate the compression forces acting on the joint. No appreciable separation of the articular surfaces occurs. It is used in the treatment of pain in a joint.

• Traction II: Sufficient force is applied to take up the "slack" or looseness of the soft tissue structures, but not to stretch them. Grade II traction can also be used for the relief of pain.

• Traction III: Soft tissues are stretched and thus this grade is described as traction-mobilization.

Gliding Translatoric gliding occurs between two joint surfaces. The term describes the movement that occurs when a bone is passively displaced in a direction **parallel** to the joint line (treatment plane). Traction I is given prior to and during gliding.

There are two grades of glides. The **first grade** involves movement of the bone, parallel to the treatment plane, to the point where the slack is taken up and the tissues become taut. The **second grade** of gliding goes beyond the stage where the slack has been taken up to the point where the tissues are stretched, and it is this second grade that is used most often when mobilizing joints.

The descriptive word "translatoric" is usually eliminated and we simply refer to movements as either traction or glides.

Maitland's Oscillatory Movements These are oscillatory movements that are performed at the rate of 2 to 3 per second (Maitland, 1986).

There are four grades of movement that can be described in relation to a straight line, representing the available range of motion. The grades relate to both accessory and physiological movements (Figure 1-1a). The movements can be modified, and an example of this modification, using the Grade II movement (Figure 1-1b) is described.

A movement that commences near the beginning of range, overlapping Grade I and the beginning of Grade II, is described as Grade II−. A movement starting deep into range and taken beyond the limit of Grade II, but not to the end of range, is described as Grade II+.

Similarly, Grades III and IV movements also adopt the plus or minus sign. If they nudge gently at the end of range, they would be considered minus grades and plus grades if there is vigorous movement at the end of range.

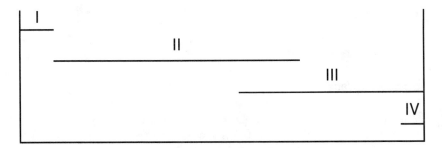

I
II
III
IV
Available Range of Motion

Grade I Small amplitude performed at the beginning of range
Grade II Large amplitude performed within the range, but not reaching the end of range
Grade III Large amplitude movement performed to limit of range
Grade IV Small amplitude at the limit of range

Figure 1-1a. Maitland's grades of movement. (Adapted from Maitland, 1986.)

II
II-
II+
Available Range of Motion

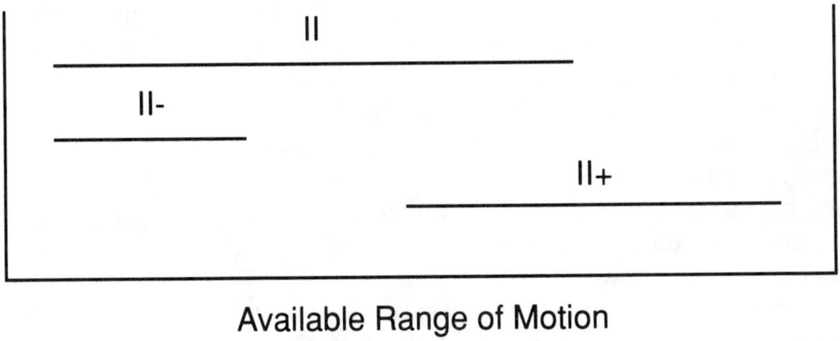

Figure 1-1b. Modification of Maitland's grade II movement. (Adapted from Maitland, 1986.)

Therapeutic Use of the Different Grades of Movement Grades I and II are used for the treatment of pain. Grades III and IV are used for increasing the range of motion in a hypomobile joint.

Arthrokinematics

Articular Surfaces

Engineers classify the convex surface as the male surface and the concave surface as the female surface. Every synovial joint contains at least one "mating pair" of articular surfaces, that is, one **male (convex)** and one **female (concave)**. When there is only one mating pair of articular surfaces, the joint is a **simple** one. A **compound** joint is one in which there is more than one mating pair. The presence of an intra-articular disc makes the joint a **complex** one. Sometimes one bone will articulate with two others, for example, the lower end of the radius with the scaphoid and the lunate. The lower end of the radius has two concave surfaces to accommodate the convex surface of the scaphoid and that of the lunate. Thus, we have two mating pairs forming the radio-scaphoid articulation and radio-lunate articulation.

Convex-Concave Rule

The convex-concave rule (Kaltenborn, 1989) can be implemented to determine in which direction, within a hypomobile joint, there is decreased gliding. Earlier it was stated that concave articular surfaces were described as female, and convex articular surfaces were described as male. Simply applied, the convex-concave rule states that a **concave** articular surface glides in the **same direction** as the distal end of the bone, and a **convex** male articular surface glides in the **opposite direction** to the bone (the male is contrary).

For example, consider a restriction of gliding at the 2nd metacarpophalangeal joint, such that flexion at the joint is limited. During the assessment, the patient's hand is supported with the palm facing down. Glides performed passively in a direction toward the palmar surface of the hand are described as "volar glides." Those glides performed in a direction toward the back or dorsum of the hand are termed "dorsal glides."

The restriction to gliding of the proximal end of the phalanx is found to be in a volar direction. This is to be expected since the articular surface is concave (female), and we know that the glide of the female surface is in the same direction as the distal end of the bone if it was free to move.

Close Packed and Loose Packed Positions

In testing for the accessory or joint play previously described, a knowledge of the close packed and loose packed positions of the joint is necessary (Table 1-1).

A joint is said to be in a **close packed** position when the articular surfaces are at the greatest degree of congruence, the ligaments are taut, and the articular surfaces cannot be separated by distraction. Any other position of the joint is called the **loose packed** position.

Table 1-1. Loose packed and close packed positions of joints

JOINT	LOOSE PACKED POSITION	CLOSE PACKED POSITION
Shoulder	Semiabduction	Abduction + lateral rotation
Ulnohumeral	Semiflexion	Extension
Radiohumeral	Extension supination	Semiflexion + semipronation
Wrist	Semiflexion	Dorsiflexion
Metacarpophalangeal (2-5)	Semiflexion + ulnar deviation	Full flexion
Interphalangeal (fingers)	Semiflexion	Extension
First carpometacarpal	Neutral position of thumb	Full opposition
Hip	Semiflexion	Extension + medial rotation
Knee	Semiflexion	Full extension
Ankle	Neutral position	Dorsiflexion
Tarsal joints	Semipronation	Full supination
Metatarsophalangeal	Neutral position	Dorsiflexion
Interphalangeal (toes)	Semiflexion	Dorsiflexion
Vertebral	Neutral position	Extension

Adapted from *Gray's Anatomy* (36th ed.), 1980.

The maximum loose packed or resting position for a joint is the one in which the joint capsule has the greatest capacity. It is the position in which joints are immobilized and the position assumed by patients when they want to "rest" a painful joint. When testing for accessory movements, it follows that the joint must not be in the close packed position since movement is not possible in this position. Instead, accessory movements are tested in the loose packed or resting position.

Descriptors of Joint Sounds

When moving peripheral joints, the therapist will often feel or hear unusual joint sounds which may or may not indicate pathology. Cyriax (1982) describes well the "snaps, clicks, cracks and crepitus."

Snaps

These are usually caused by a tendon catching against a bony prominence and then slipping over it, (e.g., long head of biceps at the shoulder, peroneal tendons at the ankle joint). Less common causes of a **pathological** nature are:

- An osteoma may first declare itself by catching against a tendon.
- A semimembranous bursa may snap as it jumps from one side of the tendon to the other, as the knee is flexed.
- Trigger finger, caused by constriction of a flexor fibrous sheath and swelling of the finger flexor tendon, releases into extension with a snap.

Clicks

Laxity of ligaments enable a bone to click as it moves in relation to its fellow bone. Clicking is common in joints unsupported by muscles (e.g., acromioclavicular [A/C] joint). It also occurs in the patellofemoral joint on extension of the knee. The latter often clicks on extension of a normal knee.

Cracks

When traction is applied to a joint, cracks occur. Synovial fluid found in joint cavities contains 15% gas, and the crack is thought to be caused by a bubble of gas collapsing.

Crepitus

Crepitus is a grating that can often be heard or felt during movement. Fine crepitus means slight roughening of the cartilaginous surfaces; coarse crepitus is due to considerable fragmentation.

CONCEPTS OF PAIN

Mechanism of Pain

The nociceptive system is responsible for pain production. Under normal circumstances this system is inactive, or relatively so, and we go about our activities in a false state of tranquillity. We are oblivious to the numerous happenings that could occur to trigger the free nerve endings of the nociceptor system. The free nerve endings of this system are found everywhere in the body (e.g., in the skin, subcutaneous tissues, capsules, ligaments), and are particularly sensitive to tissue dysfunction. Some structures are more densely supplied than others, and there is a wide distribution. Thus it is extremely difficult to selectively test individual components, say of a spinal segment, and state, with any appreciable degree of credibility, that a particular structure is at fault. It is possible, however, to identify the segment at fault, and analysis of additional information enables us to formulate hypotheses regarding the particular structure.

Mechanical forces such as pressure increases, distractions, and so on, that are sufficient to damage, stress, or deform tissues, increase the afferent activity of the nociceptor system, and pain could result. Similarly, chemical substances are also capable of enhancing the afferent activity. It is not necessary for pathology to be present for pain to be produced. Abnormal stress on normal tissue frequently produces pain. Another pain-causing combination is normal stress on abnormal tissue.

Fortunately, activity in the nociceptor system can be modified by ongoing activity in other systems. One such system is the mechanoreceptor system. Stimulation of this system can inhibit pain production; consequently, this concept is widely applied in physiotherapy treatment (e.g., massage, passive movements, electrotherapeutic modalities, and so on).

Descriptors of Pain

The therapist will find it useful to have descriptions of the different types of pain experienced by the patient; the most common and confusing of these is referred pain.

Referred Pain

This is experienced by the patient at a site distal to the location of its source; it has been described by Cyriax (1982) as an error of perception and he explains it by relating it to segmental development.

Segmental Development At about the age of one month the fetus divides into about 40 segments, the last 10 of which go into the formation of the coccyx. All but two of these disappear. The spinal segments are identified by a letter and a number, for example, C2 refers to the second cervical segment and T6 refers to the sixth thoracic segment. Similarly L3 refers to the third lumbar segment and S1 refers to the first sacral segment. Shortly after the division into segments has taken place, each segment becomes differentiated into dermatome (skin), myotome (muscles and associated soft tissues), and sclerotome (structures associated with joints, e.g., capsule, ligaments, periosteum). The upper segments are drawn upward as the head and neck develop and outward as the limbs develop. In so doing, segments C4-T2 (segments from the fourth cervical to the second thoracic) are drawn out to form the upper limb and those from L1-S3 (segments from the first lumbar to the third sacral) are drawn out to form the lower limb.

Significance of Dermatome, Myotome, and Sclerotome The dermatome of C5, the myotome of C5, and the sclerotome of C5 develop from the C5 segment, and any structure within the C5 segment (e.g., muscle, nerve root, capsule, and so on) can refer pain to the C5 dermatome. The structure may refer pain along the entire length of the dermatome or only part of it. It follows, then, that if a patient is complaining of pain in the C5 dermatome, the structure at fault will be found within the C5 segment. The dermatomes for the cervical segments and upper three thoracic segments are shown in Figures 1-2, 1-3, 1-4, and 1-5.

Types of Referred Pain Referred pain arising from a particular segment is usually described as nerve root pain (radicular) or

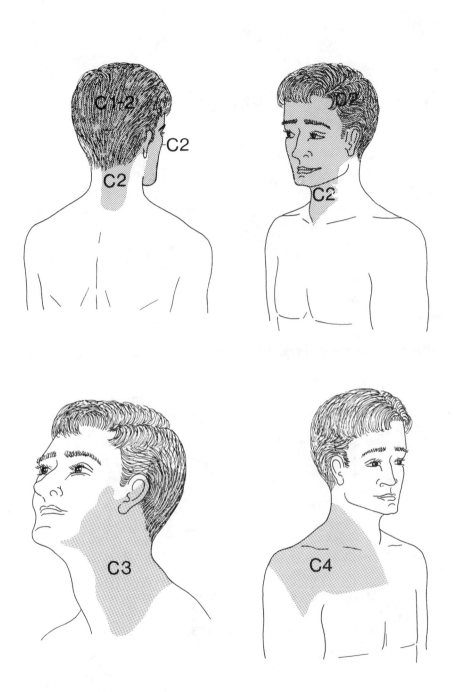

Figure 1-2. Dermatomes for C1 to C4 nerve roots.

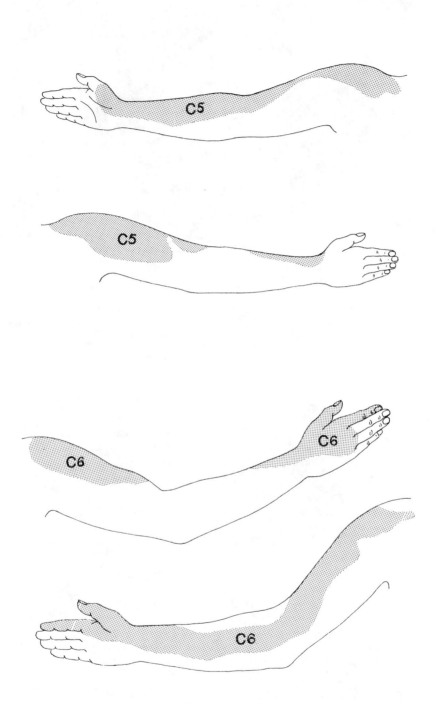

Figure 1-3. Dermatomes for C5 to C6 nerve roots.

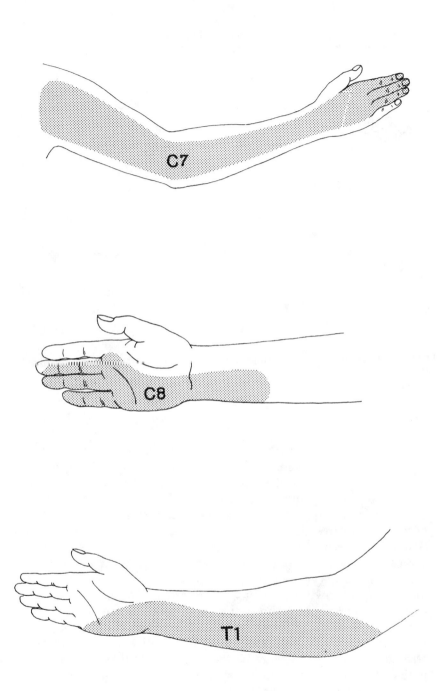

Figure 1-4. Dermatomes for C7, C8, and T1 nerve roots.

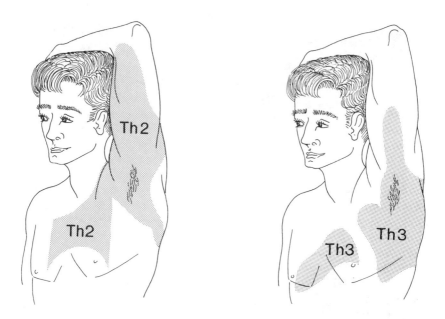

Figure 1-5. Dermatomes for Th2 and Th3 nerve roots.

somatic pain (that which arises from any structure within the musculoskeletal system except the nerve root). The type of radicular pain produced by nerve root "compression" has been described by Bogduk & Twomey (1987) as lancinating or shooting in quality and traveling within a confined area. It is accompanied by distal paresthesia, numbness, or weakness. Somatic referred pain is quite different in quality in that it is a dull ache, often severe, and diffuse in nature. In identifying the course of nerve root pain, the patient will tend to run the index finger down the course of reference; when identifying somatic referred pain, the patient will tend to use the palmar surface of the hand indicating that it is not so easy to localize. Pain is generally referred in a distal direction, thus the structure at fault is usually located proximal to where the patient feels the pain. When a structure within a segment refers pain to the corresponding dermatome it is known as *segmental reference.*

Certain structures radiate pain or paresthesia in a characteristic manner that is readily recognizable. Pressure on the dural sleeve of the nerve root refers severe pain along the whole or part of the dermatome, pressure on the nerve root alone produces distal paresthesia in the related dermatome (pins and needles) (Cyriax, 1982). Pressure on a peripheral nerve or nerve trunk produces distal paresthesia in the area related to its cutaneous supply. Superficial structures are more readily identified as the structure at fault than deep structures. There are certain structures, viz. the spinal cord and parts of the duramater that do not follow this order of reference. Instead, symptoms are referred in a bizarre and apparently unrelated way to various parts of the body. This phenomenon is described as *extrasegmental reference.*

Visceral Referred Pain The therapist should bear in mind that an organ developed from a given segment may refer pain to the dermatome corresponding to its segmental derivation, as indicated in the following list (Cyriax, 1982).

Viscera	Segmental Derivations
1. Diaphragm	C3 - 4
2. Heart	C8 - T4
3. Lungs	T2 - 5
4. Stomach and duodenum	T6 - 8
5. Liver and gall bladder	T7 - 8 right
6. Pancreas	T8 - left
7. Small intestine	T9 - 10
8. Colonic flexure	T10 - L1
9. Bladder fundus, kidney, and uterine fundus	T11 - L1
10. Colonic flexure	L2 - L3
11. Sigmoid colon and rectum	S2 - 5
12. Neck of bladder	S2 - 5
13. Prostate and urethra	S2 - 5

Other Aspects of Pain Grieve (1981) describes other aspects of pain; some of these are discussed below.

Night pain   during the night, daytime occupational, emotional, and intellectual activies are absent. Consequently, the

	modulation arising from the cerebral cortex is reduced and the patient is much more aware of pain than during the day.
Throbbing diffuse pain	vascular congestion
Bone pain	very painful and localized
Shooting pain	provoked in upper or lower limb by a cough or a sneeze and adding to existing nerve root pain due to sudden distention of vertebral veins directly caused by the rise in intrathoracic and intraabdominal pressure
Momentary catch or jab	due to disturbance of joint mechanics during a movement (i.e., joint derangement or instability)
Burning pain	can be due to chemical irritation or disruption of normal sympathetic activity; frequently accompanies syndromes exhibiting hypermobility
Vague tingling	possible circulatory disturbance. If this is so, there will be temperature and color changes in the distal part of the limb.

Concept of Joint Irritability

In addition to obtaining a profile of the pain (e.g., location, duration, and so on), we can also obtain information regarding "joint irritability" as described by Maitland (1986). Essentially the degree of irritability of a joint can be determined by **asking questions relating to factors that increase the pain and how long the increased intensity lasts.** If, for example, a simple activity like putting on a coat greatly increases the patient's pain and the increased pain lasts for several hours before subsiding, then the joint would be described as extremely irritable. The increase in pain and the length of time it lasts are out of proportion to the simplicity of the activity that aggravated it. On the other hand, if the patient's pain increased when chopping down a tree, but subsided a short time after ceasing the activity, the joint would be described as nonirritable or only mildly so.

The concept of joint irritability has great significance in both the assessment procedure to be discussed in Chapter 3 and in treatment. Evidence of severe irritability indicates that we must proceed with caution, utilizing only the gentlest of approaches of short duration in both assessment and treatment. Other signs of joint irritability are pain at rest, disturbances of sleep, inability to sleep on the affected side, and the extent to which the pain radiates. Other important factors relate to whether the pain is constant or intermittent. If a patient is in constant pain, the joint is considered more irritable than if the patient experiences intermittent pain. When questioned regarding the constant or intermittent nature of their pain patients will frequently state that their pain is constant. However, when asked: "Are there 5 minutes during the day when you do not have pain?" they will give a positive response; this means that their pain is intermittent and less irritable than they had first indicated.

SUMMARY

In this chapter, the concepts of joint movement were described including physiological, accessory, translatoric, and oscillatory movements. The concave-convex rule, and the close packed and loose packed positions were defined. An interpretation was provided for the joint sounds; pain was introduced in terms of its mechanism and descriptors, and referred pain was discussed in terms of radicular pain, somatic referred pain, and viscerogenic referred pain. Finally, the concept of joint irritability was introduced.

CHAPTER 2

The Use of Movement in the Assessment Process

STRUCTURES THAT CAUSE PAIN

So far, we have learned how to identify the segment accommodating the structure at fault and certain elements of the peripheral nervous system within that segment that may be responsible for the patient's discomfort. There are, however, numerous other structures contained in a segment that can cause pain. Structures can be divided into either contractile structures or inert structures. Contractile structures are: (a) muscle, (b) tendon, and (c) tenoperiosteal insertion.

Strictly speaking, tendons are not contractile, but lesions of tendons behave as if they are in their response to muscle contraction, that is, they cause pain. It is for this reason that they are listed under contractile structures. Inert structures are noncontractile and consist of: (a) ligaments, (b) bursae, and (c) capsules.

To identify whether a structure at fault is contractile or inert, Cyriax (1982) devised the *Theory of Selective Tension*. Briefly stated, this theory postulates that when tension is applied to an injured contractile or inert structure it will cause pain. A **contractile** tissue lesion will cause pain when the corresponding muscle **contracts**, and an **inert** tissue lesion will cause pain when the structure containing the lesion is **stretched.**

Isometric Resisted Contractions

By utilizing isometric resisted contractions, it is possible to identify the muscle group containing the disabled member, since pain will be produced when resistance is applied to that particular muscle group. For example, resisted isometric abduction will cause pain if there is a lesion of one of the abductors. Similarly, if the problem lies with one of the lateral rotators, resisted isometric lateral rotation will cause pain. Since no joint movement occurs, the fault in both cases must be located in a contractile structure. Resisted isometric contractions also inform us about the quality of the nerve conduction, which is determined by the strength of the muscular response. This aspect will be discussed later.

Passive Movements

These movements are utilized to detect lesions in inert structures since the latter will be subjected to stretch when the joint is moved passively, and thus cause pain.

Relationship of Pain to Resistance

During the performance of a passive movement on a joint containing an inert lesion, three possibilities arise:

1. Pain can develop before resistance to movement is detected by the therapist. This is indicative of an acute situation, for example, inflammation in the first stage of healing. Under these circumstances the therapist would proceed with great care, if at all.
2. Pain can appear at the same time that resistance is detected and, in the stages of healing, this would correspond to the subacute stage in the healing process. Consequently, the therapist would proceed gently with the examination.

3. Pain may appear after the therapist has detected resistance, in which case the lesion would probably be in the chronic stage of healing, and the therapist can proceed with more vigor.

Active Movements

During the performance of an active movement muscle contraction occurs, and inert structures are stretched because joint movement also occurs. Thus, pain occurring during the performance of an active movement could be due to a lesion in either a contractile or an inert structure or both. Without further testing, it is difficult to differentiate between the two. However, active movements do indicate the following:

- the range of available movement
- the willingness of the patient to move
- the patient has sufficient strength to perform the movement either weakly or strongly

Summary

At this stage in the assessment process the following information may be revealed:

1. The segment containing the lesion at fault (from a knowledge of dermatome distribution).
2. A contractile structure is at fault (from the painful response to resisted isometric contraction).
3. An inert structure is at fault (from the response to passive movements) and the severity of the lesion is evident (from the relationship between pain and resistance to movement).
4. The state of the nerve conduction is apparent (from the response to resisted isometric contractions).

It should be noted that where a resisted isometric contraction causes pain, a weak response may be due to that and not to the quality of nerve conduction. In some instances, however, patients are able to match the therapist's resistance with a strong isometric contraction, even in the presence of pain.

Additional Diagnostic Findings and Their Significance

In addition to the findings from the various movement tests just described, there are other findings from the examination process which are helpful to the therapist. Pain may appear during an arc of movement; the sensation beneath the therapist's hand during a passive movement may feel abnormal when compared to the patient's other side, or the restriction of motion may be in a predictable pattern. These and other findings are explained below.

Painful Arc

This finding indicates that a tender structure is being squeezed between two bony structures, or one bony structure and another structure. It is characterized by a part of the range being pain free, followed by a painful part of the range, and followed again by a pain free range. It is a common finding in problems associated with the glenohumeral joint.

End Feel

At the end of the available passive range of motion the therapist's hand will experience different sensations. For example, the sensation may be springy or it may be an abrupt halt. There are normal end feels that are experienced when the joint is free of pathology and abnormal end feels that occur in the presence of pathology in the joint. The normal and abnormal end feels are described below.

Normal End Feels

Under normal circumstances, the sensation beneath the therapist's hand at the end of the passive range of motion will be one of following:

- *Bone to Bone:* A sudden halt to movement, for example, on extension of the elbow.
- *Capsular Feel:* Hard arrest of movement with some give; for example, this feel is evident when the extreme range of lateral rotation at the normal shoulder or hip is reached.

- *Tissue Approximation:* Normal sensation felt at full passive flexion of a normal elbow or knee.

Note: Sometimes a definite end feel is not discernable due to tension in the antagonistic muscle group. Under such circumstances the sensation imparted to the therapist's hand would be soft tissue stretch.

Abnormal End Feels

The abnormal end feels are those that are found in the presence of joint pathology. They are empty end feel, spasm, springy block, and abnormal capsular feel.

- *Empty End Feel:* Sometimes a passive movement can be very painful for the patient, and yet the therapist is not at the end of the available range, that is, there is no restricting sensation. This lack of sensation beneath the therapist's hand is called an empty end feel. The pain experienced by the patient often results in his or her requesting that the therapist curtail the movement before resistance is felt.
- *Spasm:* In the presence of acute or subacute arthritis a passive movement may be stopped by muscle spasm suddenly coming into play in which case the therapist will experience a firm end feel.
- *Springy Block:* Visible rebound is felt at the end of the available range of motion. This is usually indicative of an intraarticular block or derangement. An example of this would be a meniscus problem in the knee which blocks extension.
- *Abnormal Capsular Feel:* This imparts a similar sensation to the normal capsular end feel except it appears before the normal end of range is reached.

Capsular Patterns

This is a characteristic proportional restriction of motion within a specific joint due to involvement of the synovial membrane or the capsule. Under these circumstances, every shoulder will present with the same proportional restriction, as will every hip joint, although the characteristic pattern will differ from that of the shoulder. Other movements of the joint may also be restricted, but as long as the the movements characterizing the proportional restriction for the particular joint are present the capsular pattern is exhibited.

There is some discrepancy in the literature regarding capsular patterns (Magee, 1987). The following patterns are largely based on Cyriax (1982) who was the first person to define them. They are listed in order of the severity of restriction for each joint.

Temporomandibular joint	restriction in mouth opening
Cervical spine	rotation and side flexion equally limited; extension somewhat limited; flexion full range, but painful
Glenohumeral joint	lateral rotation exhibits the greatest degree of limitation, then abduction, and finally medial rotation, which exhibits the least limitation
Humeroulnar joint	more limitation of flexion than extension
Upper radioulnar joint	equal limitation of pronation and supination
Lower radioulnar joint	full range of motion with pain at both extremes of rotation
Wrist	equal degree of limitation of flexion and extension
1st carpometacarpal	limitation of abduction and joint extension; full flexion
Thumb and fingers	more restriction of flexion than extension
Hip joint	gross limitation of flexion abduction and medial rotation, slight limitation of extension
Knee joint	gross limitation of flexion (e.g., 90°), slight limitation of extension (5-10°)
Ankle joint	more limitation of plantar flexion than dorsi flexion (calf muscles are assumed to be normal length)

Talocalcaneum joint	limitation of varus range
1st Metatarsophalan-geal joint	marked limitation of extension, slight limitation of flexion

Noncapsular Patterns

Noncapsular patterns are found in joints that do not exhibit a proportional restriction of motion and, therefore, are not arthritic. Examples of joint problems exhibiting a noncapsular pattern of motion are ligamentous adhesions that may result in restriction of motion in one direction only, and intraarticular disorders such as loose bodies or disc lesions that will result in a restriction of motion other than that exhibited by the capsular pattern.

Common Causes of Noncapsular Patterns in Specific Joints

Cervical spine	internal derangement due to disc fragment
Glenohumeral joint	acute subdeltoid bursitis
Elbow	loose body
Inferior radioulnar joint	mal-union of Colles fracture
Wrist	subluxation of capitate bone
Hip joint	bursitis or loose body
Knee joint	meniscus or loose body

PALPATION

This is an art and, as such, requires practice to achieve. It is one of the most important aspects of examination and yet is frequently done hastily and without much thought. Findings may be few, and those that are elicited may be incorrectly interpreted. Concentration and a quiet environment are necessary ingredients in the development of palpatory skill. Chatty conversation, which usually takes place during laboratory sessions, should be eliminated in order to detect slight changes in texture, shape, structure, and so forth. The therapist must focus solely on what is being felt beneath the pads of the fingers, the palmar surface of the hand and fingers, or the dorsal aspect of the hand. Only the degree of pressure necessary for detection is applied.

Greenwood (1989) has reported on three different aspects in the development of the palpatory sense. The first is reception when the stimulation of the tissues being palpated is received by the proprioceptors and mechanoreceptors of the hand. The second and third aspects are transmission and interpretation when the impulses received are transmitted via the peripheral and central system to the brain where they are analyzed and interpreted.

The Significance of Palpatory Skills

Palpatory skills are used for the following purposes:

- to detect abnormality in the texture of tissues
- to detect both visual and tactile asymmetry
- to detect differences in movement and quality throughout the range of motion and the type of end feel on completion of the available range
- to detect any change in the palpatory findings over time.

Greenwood (1989) suggests the use of paired descriptions for the structures being palpated, for example, moist-dry, painful-nonpainful, circumscribed-diffuse, and so on. In addition, he recommends the use of a scale to measure the normality, or severity of the abnormality, of the tissues being palpated.

Parts of the Hand Utilized in Palpation

Moving distally to proximally, the following parts of the hand are used in palpation.

1. The pads of the fingers, which are extremely sensitive, are used with very gentle pressure to detect changes in texture and tension of the more superficial structures (e.g., skin).
2. The palmar surface of the metacarpals, which are sensitive to vibration and changes in the degree of moisture.
3. The palmar aspect of the hand is used to detect and recognize gross shapes.
4. The dorsal aspect of the hand is generally used to detect changes in temperature.

The therapist must learn to use each part of the hand gently and slowly. Only then will she or he be able to detect subtle changes in texture or temperature of the tissue being palpated. The softness of skin and the firmness of bone should be noted.

Skin

This forms the external surface of the body and is highly sensitive. Its many functions include minimizing the harmful effects of a variety of stresses, for example, thermal and chemical, as well taking part in heat control and providing a protective barrier to invading organisms. Much can be learned from its mobility, temperature, texture, and so on.

Mobility The therapist should move the skin gently over subcutaneous tissues noting the smoothness of the movement. She or he should attempt to compare the feeling detected with the feeling sensed over scar tissue. The change in textures should be noted. The pads of the fingers can be moved over the hair on the skin and that sensation noted.

Temperature With the dorsum of the hand, one should be able to detect changes in temperature. At first, the hand is a small distance away from the tissue being tested. The skin temperature can be compared with the temperature of the table top. Next, the hand is placed on the skin and moved gently along the skin surface to pick up temperature changes. Cool areas may be due to decreased vascularity. The detection of heat indicates increased vascularity and when felt over a lesion means that the lesion is in an active stage (i.e., stage of healing). Heat is felt over the site of a broken bone or a ligamentous sprain and remains as long as the healing stage continues. Bleeding into a joint (hemarthrosis) is always accompanied by heat.

Moisture Increased moisture of the skin can be due to an increase in sympathetic activity in the area, or to an increase in vascularity. Dry, scaly skin may be due to a decrease in sympathetic activity.

Subcutaneous Tissues The therapist should try to distinguish the feel of the subcutaneous fat from that of the skin. Pressure should not be progressively harder, but rather applied gently enough to make the distinction. The feel of blood vessels may be determined; next, the feel of a muscle at its broadest part. One should ask how it feels compared to the skin and subcutaneous fat. The fingers are moved onto a tendon and the sensation beneath the fingers is registered. The differences between tendon and ligament are noted. Finally, one notes the hard resistance of bone.

Palpating for Tenderness Eliciting tenderness on deep palpation can be a very misleading symptom and by itself is unreliable. This is because deep somatic tissues can refer tenderness on palpation and frequently the tender area does not correspond to the site of the lesion. However, tenderness associated with superficial lesions (e.g., tendons, ligaments, and so on) generally does correspond to the site of the lesion. Tenderness on palpation, then, has a confirmatory value in terms of identifying a superficial structure at fault.

SUMMARY

In this chapter, the utilization of active movement, passive stretch, and isometric contraction within the musculoskeletal system have been described. The relationship between pain and resistance to movement provided additional information relating to joint irritability. Normal and abnormal end feels, and capsular and noncapsular patterns were defined. The importance of palpation and the use of different parts of the hand in the palpatory process were discussed.

CHAPTER 3

The Clinical Examination

The clinical examination consists of two parts: a subjective examination and an objective examination.

The Subjective Examination

Before describing the component parts of the subjective examination it is well to consider the optimum conditions under which this will take place. Benjamin (1969) has pointed out that an atmosphere conducive to communication without distraction is important (Figure 3-1). The next stage is to establish rapport with the patient. The word "rapport" is often interpreted as meaning indulging in small talk, but it means much more. Rapport is an harmonious, cooperative interaction between the patient and the health care professional (Bernstein, Bernstein, & Dana, 1974). It involves making the patient feel welcome, comfortable, and demonstrating a real interest in the patient and the patient's problems. Patients are naturally apprehensive and time taken initially to create a meaningful and relaxing environment is time well spent.

During the subjective part of the clinical examination, the patient is encouraged to relate to the therapist the following information relating to his or her *current* problem:

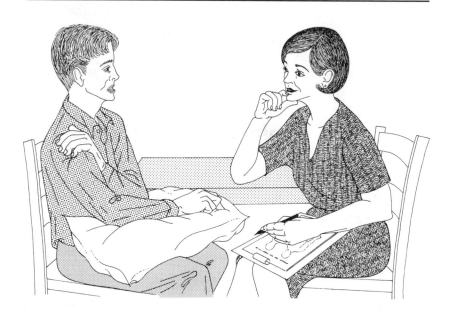

Figure 3-1. The subjective examination "Listen to the patient!"

- age, marital state, ages of children (if any), occupation
- where the patient feels the dominant pain (P1) that caused him or her to seek help
- length of time the pain has been present (onset)
- what happens to the pain under given circumstances (behavior of the problem)
- information as above regarding other pains (i.e., P2, P3, and so on).

The type of information obtained in the subjective examination is based largely on what the patient feels, that is, symptoms. The therapist utilizes the interviewing process to gain this information, and the most important initial step is to establish good rapport with the patient.

It is the responsibility of the therapist to gently control the questioning process and to gain all the relevant information in the shortest possible time. To achieve this, the patient must have the examiner's undivided attention. This involves not only attending physically to the patient, but observing and listening as well. The patient's body language, in terms of posture, willingness to move, and facial expression can be very informative. To ensure that the patient has the therapist's undivided attention, every effort must be made to ensure that interruptions are avoided, or at least cut to the absolute minimum.

In initiating a pattern of question and answer the examiner implies that he or she is the authority. This hardly contributes to the establishment of rapport discussed previously. Since questions need to be asked, the following points should be considered:

- The questions about to be asked should be challenged on the basis of the value of the information obtained. Unnecessary questions should be avoided.
- The therapist should remain aware that he or she is asking the questions.
- The therapist must be sensitive to the questions asked by the patient, whether or not those questions are asked outright.

Maitland (1986) has pointed out that communication between two people is not easy under normal circumstances. Therfore, he recommends adhering to a certain format regarding questions.

Guidelines for Asking Questions

Questions should be organized and asked:

- with a specific purpose in mind
- from a sound knowledge base, so that the answer can be interpreted correctly and the therapist knows which question to ask next
- in layman's language, which the patient can understand
- briefly and to the point
- one question at a time
- phrased in a way that avoids leading the patient.

Following is a scenario incorporating the points just mentioned.

Subjective Examination Scenario

For the sake of clarity and comprehension, the patient selected is ideal — her answers are direct and to the point.

Q.1. "What has brought you in to see me today?"
A. "My right shoulder is painful."

Q.2. "Can you show me where you feel the pain?"
A. "Here." (The patient places her fingers on her right shoulder then moves them down her arm to below her elbow.)

Q.3. "Is the pain there all the time?"
A. "Yes."

Q.4. "Is there any time during the day when you are free of pain?" (This is a pursuing question relating to question 3.)
A. "Not that I am aware of."

Q.5. "Can you describe the pain for me. Is it tingling, stabbing, burning, or a dull ache?"
(Note the avoidance of a leading question here.)
A. "A dull ache."

Q.6. "How would you rate your pain on a scale of 1 to 10, where 1 is the smallest amount of pain and 10 is the most severe?"
A. "Seven."

Q.7. "Does the pain disturb your sleep?"
A. "Yes."

Q.8. "Can you sleep on the right side?"
A. "No."

Q.9. "What makes your pain worse?"
A. "Ironing. If I iron for 10 minutes my arm gets really sore and I have to stop."

Q.10. "How long does the increased pain last?"
A. "Over an hour if I do not take Tylenol."

Q.11. "Other than Tylenol, what eases your pain?"
A. "Rubbing my shoulder and using a heating pad."

In this scenario, the therapist is focusing on the patient's current history, that is, events relating to her painful right shoulder. The therapist records all the information obtained from the patient, utilizing a body chart to describe the characteristics of the patient's pain.

Interpreting the Patient's Answers

The answers to questions 2 and 3 tell the therapist that the patient's problem is severe because of its spatial (extending down below the elbow) and temporal (constant pain) qualities. The response to question 5 gives the therapist some idea of the structure at fault. Answers to questions 6, 7, 8, 9, and 10 indicate to the therapist that the lesion is irritable (see Chapter 1), which means he or she should proceed cautiously with the objective examination to avoid exacerbating the condition. Indeed in some instances it may be prudent to postpone the objective examination until the danger of exacerbation has passed.

What other questions need to be asked? It is conceivable that the patient may have a coexisting condition, such as an intermittent backache (P2). While this may not be all that troublesome, the therapist would need to address questions similar to those outlined in the scenario, to this problem also. Information regarding medication is of vital importance when planning a treatment program. The patient's age can be a helpful indicator, since certain conditions tend to develop within certain age groups. Knowledge of the patient's occupation and hobbies is helpful in determining whether the condition is being further irritated and also in treatment planning. When all questions regarding the patient's current history have been asked, the therapist proceeds with questions pertaining to the patient's past history. Of particular interest would be information that might account for, or relate to, the patient's present condition. Finally there are certain mandatory questions that must be asked. These are categorized under the headings of medication, dizziness, spinal cord signs, general health, and past medical history.

Medication It is important to note if the patient is on anticoagulants. This type of medication may produce hemarthrosis, particularly if the patient has to undergo vigorous physiotherapy.

The patient may be on analgesics or antiinflammatory medication. Both tend to mask the seriousness of the condition. Corticosteroid medication can cause osteoporosis.

Dizziness Dizziness can be an indication of vertebral artery insufficiency or a disturbance in the inner ear. A differential test(s) needs to be performed to determine the cause.

Spinal Cord Signs These tend to manifest themselves in the form of an unsteady gait or weakness of the lower limbs.

General Health and Past Medical History It is important to know whether the patient has had any inflammatory conditions such as rheumatoid arthritis. Inflammatory conditions can weaken the ligaments of joints causing instability.

Carcinoma can metastasize in bones, so it is important to know whether the patient has had cancer and whether they are experiencing severe bone pain. Radiotherapy can cause osteoporosis in the surrounding bone tissue.

On completion of the subjective examination, the experienced clinician will be able to detect certain patterns and to link one piece of information with another when analyzing the patient's responses. However, it is only when all the information from the objective examination has been recorded and analyzed that meaningful hypotheses can be formulated regarding the patient's problem. The objective examination will be considered next.

THE OBJECTIVE EXAMINATION

This part of the examination is concerned with what the therapist observes and with the findings which are elicited from various movements and tests.

The objective examination can be divided into a scan examination and a detailed examination.

The Scan Examination

During the scan, the upper or lower quadrant of the body, depending on the location of pain, will be subjected to a quick examination to determine the specific area containing the lesion at fault. For instance, if the patient is experiencing pain in the forearm or hand, an upper quadrant scan will be performed. This involves:

- a quick examination of the cervical spine
- passive tests for the peripheral joints of the upper limb
- isometric testing of the myotomes to determine the integrity of nerve root conduction

- testing the reflexes associated with the upper limb
- sensory testing of the dermatomes associated with the upper quadrant.

If the patient is experiencing pain in the knee, a lower quadrant scan will be performed involving the lumbar spine, peripheral joints of the lower limb, myotomes, reflexes, and dermatomes associated with the lower quadrant. The scan examinations are described in detail in Chapters 4 and 8.

The Detailed Examination

Once the *area at fault* has been determined, from an analysis of the information gained from the scan, that area is subjected to a detailed examination to determine the *structure at fault*. If an upper quadrant scan was used, the detailed examination could be performed on the cervical spine, or any of the peripheral joints of the upper limb.

COMPONENT PARTS OF THE OBJECTIVE EXAMINATION

The objective examination consists of four parts: (1) observation, (2) functional testing, (3) sensory and reflex testing, and (4) palpation.

Observation

Observation is a continuous process. The patient is observed as he or she enters the department, positions her- or himself, and throughout the subjective examination. The therapist watches the patient's face for signs of pain and observes the patient for signs of protective postures (e.g., hugging the arm to the side, fixed position for head and neck, and so on). In addition, the therapist is continually searching for signs that may contribute to, or be the cause of, the patient's problem.

Close attention is paid to standing posture, starting with the head and neck and extending down to the feet. Bony prominences and other anatomical landmarks are observed for asymmetry as the therapist carefully compares findings on one side of the body with those on the other. Asymmetrical findings are recorded; these may or may not be significant to the patient's problem, and the therapist must be wary of assuming that every asymmetry is the cause of the patient's problem. On completion of this part of the objective examination, the signs recorded could include any, or all, of the following:

- deviations from the postural norm and the levels at which they occur
- abrasion, swelling, muscle spasm, and muscle atrophy and where they are located
- color changes, signs of increased perspiration, respiratory rate, and fatigue.

Two things need to be emphasized at this point. The first is that the signs listed are fairly common findings, some more than others; however, it is conceivable that observation could reveal very little. In this case, the therapist would have to rely on the findings in the remaining part of the objective examination, as well as the information gained from the subjective examination. Second, if the subjective examination indicates strongly that the problem lies in the upper part of the body, that is, cervical spine and upper extremity, observation would be confined to the upper part of the body. The next step in the objective examination is functional testing.

Functional Testing

This involves testing the soft tissue structure in the area where the tissue at fault is thought to be located. Active, passive, and isometric tests are used.

Active movements reveal nothing about the cause of the patient's problem, since during an active movement both joint structures and muscles are involved. It is, therefore, difficult to determine whether the patient's pain is caused by a joint that has moved or a muscle that has contracted. It is possible to pick up some useful information regarding the willingness of the patient to move, range of motion, and whether the latter is pain free. It should be noted, however, that the range of motion observed may bear little relation to the passive range. This is particularly so if there is a lesion within the prime muscle involved in the movement. Pain caused by contraction of the muscle could well be the limiting factor.

Isometric contractions utilize components of muscle only and are used to detect painful muscle responses and weakness of the muscles tested. The responses elicited and their interpretation are listed below.

Response	Interpretation
Strong contraction, no pain	Normal muscle
Strong contraction, with pain	Muscle lesion
Weak contraction with pain	Irritable muscle lesion on its own or combined with interference in the conductivity of the nerve
Weak contraction with no pain; two possibilities:	(a) interference with the conductivity of the nerve (b) old rupture of muscle tendon

As stated previously, a muscle will produce a weak response if there is interference in nerve conductivity due to pathology or trauma. The integrity of a nerve root conductivity can be tested by selecting a muscle supplied by that particular nerve root and determining the isometric strength compared with the other side. For instance, the triceps muscle is supplied by C7. If on testing that muscle there is weakness, but no pain, then interference with nerve root conductivity would be suspected. This concept is applied frequently during the objective examination. A list of muscles and their respective nerve roots is given in Chapter 4 as the various parts of the musculoskeletal system are examined.

The interpretation of the responses to isometric contraction tests, described previously, has been confined to the muscle-tendon complex or the nerve. It is important to note that pain and weakness also exist in the presence of serious underlying pathology, for example, a fracture. In this instance, the tension of the muscle over the fracture site causes sufficient pain to produce a very weak response. The therapist must always be alert to the possibility of serious underlying pathology during any testing procedure.

So far in the objective examination some information has been obtained, in a nonspecific manner, from performing active movements and in a specific manner by performing isometric tests. Next, tests will be considered that will determine the integrity of joint structures, for example, capsule, ligaments, bursae, and so on. These structures do not possess contractile capability and are therefore described as inert. They are tested by utilizing passive movements.

Passive movements are performed entirely by the therapist with no involvement of contractile structures. Consequently, signs and symptoms elicited must be due to involvement of the joint structures, that is, the inert structures. There are two exceptions to this rule.

1. Lesions in tendons can cause pain if they are squeezed during the performance of passive movements.
2. An abnormal muscle complex can give rise to pain if any part of it is stretched during the performance of a passive or active movement.

During the passive movement test, the therapist is not only trying to determine the extent of the patient's range of motion, but the cause of the restriction, if one exists. To do this, the therapist must be able to tune in to the sensation imparted to his or her hands as he or she reaches the restricted range. These sensations are commonly known as "end feels" and will be described in more detail than in Chapter 2.

End Feel As stated previously, the term "end feel" is used to describe the sensation imparted to the therapist's hands at the end of the available range of motion. Under normal circumstances, every joint exhibits some resistance at the end of range. These sensations are called "normal end feels" and will be described first.

Normal End Feels These sensations have the following characteristics.

1. *Soft tissue approximation.* This occurs when soft tissue from one part of the limb comes into contact with soft tissue from another part of the limb, thus restricting range of motion. Two good examples of soft tissue approximation occur (a) when the elbow is flexed and (b) when the knee is flexed. In both instances there is approximation of soft tissue experienced by the therapist as a soft resistance.

2. *Bone on bone.* There is a hard arrest of movement felt suddenly at the end of range when that range is restricted by the bony joint articulations coming into contact with each other. The classical example of a bone on bone end feel is extension of the elbow, where there is felt a sudden hard arrest of movement.

3. *Capsular.* Most peripheral joints impart this type of end feel. It is recognized by some initial resistance followed by a harder arrest of movement with a bounce to it. This is the sensation felt when the end of range is reached in, for example, external rotation of the shoulder.

Abnormal End Feels These sensations are comprised of the following characteristics.

1. *Abnormal capsular end feel.* This is described as abnormal because it occurs before the end of the normal range of motion of a joint due to the presence of pathology. The sensation is that of the normal capsular end feel, but the therapist experiences it at the pathological limit of range of motion rather than at the anatomical limit. It is frequently accompanied by discomfort.

2. *Springy block.* The sensation here is one of a sudden block to the movement followed immediately by a springing out of it. Again, it occurs before the anatomical limit to range of motion is reached. This type of sensation is experienced, for example, in the knee joint where the block might be due to a torn meniscus blocking movement.

3. *Spasm.* This comes into play suddenly during the performance of a passive movement, and acts protectively to prevent further movement from taking place. It can be seen, and it too imparts a hard sensation to the therapist's hand. It is usually an indication of the presence of a severe condition. The spasm may or may not be accompanied by pain.

4. *Empty sensation.* Occasionally when the examiner is using passive movements, the patient will cry out in pain and yet no resistance to movement has been felt by the examiner — there is nothing there, an empty sensation. This is found in the presence of a significant disease process, for example, neoplasm.

Special Tests In addition to the passive and isometric tests, there are special tests that may be included in the detailed examination. These tests provide the therapist with information that may confirm specific findings or elicit others.

Interpretation of the Relationship Between Pain and Resistance As discussed in Chapter 2, the relationship between pain and resistance, in terms of which appears first in the passive movement, or their appearance at the same time, provides the therapist with valuable information.

- *Pain before resistance:* When this occurs it is a warning sign to the therapist to proceed with great caution, or not to proceed at all. An acute condition is indicated.
- *Pain with resistance:* This tells the therapist that the passive movement may continue, but with caution. A subacute condition is indicated.
- *Pain following resistance:* With these findings, usually found near the end of range, the therapist can continue the examination. A chronic condition is indicated.

A consideration of the findings from the performance of passive movements not only tells the therapist what the available range of motion is, but whether it is the normal anatomical range or is limited by pathology. Further information is revealed by the type of resistance encountered, that is, end feel. Finally, the relationship between pain and resistance tells the therapist whether he or she may proceed with the examination and how careful he or she must be.

Sensory and Reflex Testing

During the subjective examination the patient may have identified an area of numbness that could infer a lesion of the sensory component of the nerve root. To confirm the presence of sensory loss, the therapist lightly runs the pads of her fingers *across* the dermatomes, starting, for example, with the side of the neck and terminating in the hand, asking the patient if any difference is noted as she does so. Additional supportive information may be obtained from testing the reflexes which could be sluggish or absent in the presence of interference in nerve root conductivity.

Palpation

This aspect was discussed in detail in Chapter 2. For a review of the information, see pages 25-28.

SUMMARY

In this chapter, guidelines have been presented for asking questions. A scenario provided an appropriate format for the subjective examination with interpretations of the patient's responses to questions. The component parts of the scan were introduced and those of the detailed examination were described fully to provide a framework for the objective assessment.

• • • • • • • •

CHAPTER 4

Upper Quadrant Scan and Detailed Examination of the Cervical Spine

UPPER QUADRANT SCREENING EXAMINATION (SCAN)

The upper quadrant consists of the cervical spine, the shoulder girdle, the glenohumeral joint, the elbow, the radio-ulnar joints, the joints of the wrist and hand, and the soft tissue and bony structures associated with these joints. The upper quadrant screening examination (scan) is a quick examination of key structures of the above joints. The structures tested are selected so that the results of the tests provide the therapist with sufficient information to identify the area in the upper quadrant that contains the structure at fault. For example, an analysis of the information obtained from the scan examination may implicate the glenohumeral joint and associated structures as the cause of the patient's problem. A detailed examination of the glenohumeral joint and its associated structures would then be carried out to identify the specific structure at fault.

The necessity of performing a scan examination may be questioned if it were not for the fact that the phenomenon of referred pain creates so much confusion in the musculoskeletal examination. In recent years the cervical spine has been identified as the cause of much of the pain experienced by patients in the upper extremity (Corrigan & Maitland, 1983; Grieve, 1981; Hoppenfeld, 1976; Maigne, 1972; Wells, 1982).

COMPONENT PARTS

Patient's Medical History

Taking a patient's medical history was described in Chapter 3. It is imperative, however, to emphasize the importance of determining at the outset the cause of a patient's complaint of dizziness, because this could be caused by vertebrobasilar arterial insufficiency (VAI).

Vertebrobasilar Arterial Insufficiency

Initially, dizziness may be the only symptom of VAI but later other symptoms such as double vision (diplopia), drop attacks, mechanical interference with speech (dysarthria), and difficulty in swallowing (dysphagia) may be part of the syndrome.

A patient may complain of dizziness when looking overhead. If this is so the therapist can place the patient in the prone position and ask the patient to extend the neck. It may be necessary to sustain the extended position for 10 seconds to reproduce the dizziness.

On the other hand, it may be that the patient's dizziness comes on when turning the head from side to side. In this case, it is necessary to distinguish between the vertebral artery and the vestibular mechanism in the inner ear as the causative factor. This can be achieved by asking the patient to sit; while the therapist firmly holds the patient's head, the patient rotates the trunk first to one side then the other. Again it may be necessary to sustain rotation before dizziness appears. The reproduction of dizziness in one or both of these tests implicates the vertebral artery. Therefore, great care should be taken when proceeding with the assessment and treatment.

Other tests to determine the cause of dizziness have been described by Grant (1988).

Observation

The various aspects regarding observation, mentioned previously, are carried out in the scan examination. However, if an upper quadrant scan examination is being performed, it is because the therapist suspects that the patient's problem lies either in the cervical spine or the upper extremity. During observation, close attention must be paid to the posture of the head, neck, and shoulder girdle. When observing the patient from the **anterior** aspect, particular note should be taken to determine whether:

- the nose and chin are in mid-line of the body
- the level of the ear lobes lie on the same line
- the level of the shoulders are equal or poking forward
- bony abnormalities of the shoulder girdle are evident
- there are changes in muscle contour.

Observation from the **lateral** aspect largely involves the head and neck position. Is there a poking chin? Is there a compensatory cervicothoracic kyphosis? Viewed from the **posterior** aspect, the following should be observed:

- the levels of the spines of the scapula
- the levels of the inferior angles of the scapula
- the position of the scapulae on the chest wall
- spinal deviations and evidence of muscle spasm

Some of the significant signs, and their interpretation, will be discussed here.

The Poking Chin

This is one of the most common postural faults. However, the secondary effects of this malady quite often escape notice. It has been pointed out (Darnell, 1983) that the poking chin sets off a chain reaction that can have deleterious effects on structures extending proximally as far as the temporomandibular joint and distally as far as the lumbar spine. In the cervical and shoulder girdle region, the anterior and lateral musculature of the cervical spine should be observed for abnormalities. In the forward head position, as seen in the patient with the poking chin, the head is situated in a more anterior position than is normal; if the lateral and anterior cervical musculature become tight the upper and middle cervical vertebrae will be pulled forward and downward. In addition, the posterior cervical muscles will contract, pulling downward on the occiput. If the situation were left as just described, the patient would lose the ability to look straight ahead. However, compensation occurs by virtue of a forward bend in the lower cervical and upper thoracic spine, producing a cervicothoracic kyphosis. This compensatory correction restores the patient's ability to look horizontally. In summary, the poking chin may well be accompanied by:

- tight anterior and lateral cervical musculature
- hyperactive posterior cervical muscles
- a cervicothoracic kyphosis.

Darnell (1983) describes a chronology of possible events, and his article is worthy of serious consideration.

Abnormal Positions of the Scapula

There are many reasons why the scapula would assume an abnormal position on the posterior chest wall. Two of these are described below.

Unilateral Elevation of the Scapula This posture is assumed by patients who complain of pain in the ipsilateral shoulder as a result of nerve root irritation, tight levator scapulae, and so on. The patient assumes this position to ease the tension in the nerve root or tight muscles. During the subjective examination, a woman patient may have indicated that the bra strap of the contralateral shoulder is always slipping down, or if a male patient wears braces to hold up his pants, he may complain that the one on the unaffected side slips down.

A Protracted Scapula A scapula abducted on the posterior chest wall may be an indication of weakness of the rhomboids. If this abnormal scapular posture remains uncorrected, traction of the suprascapular nerve may develop, with resultant weakness of the spinati. A long-established protracted scapula will also result in tightness of the pectoralis minor.

Functional Testing

The tests involved in functional testing are used to determine the quality of active movements of the cervical spine and peripheral joints, isometric contractions of selected muscles of the myotomes, reflexes, and the sensory quality of the dermatomes.

Movements of the Cervical Spine

The following movements are tested actively with the patient in the sitting position: flexion, extension, right side flexion, left side flexion, right rotation, and left rotation.

Overpressure is applied by the therapist at the end of the patient's active range, provided the range achieved by the patient is pain free. The end feel will be noted as will a painful response to the overpressure. The addition of the overpressure constitutes a passive movement, and the pain created must be caused by an inert structure.

Movements of the Peripheral Joints

The following movements, except for the first two, are performed first on the unaffected side of the body, then on the affected side, for every joint tested. The therapist performs overpressure (OP) after each movement. Differences noted between the two sides are recorded.

> *Temporomandibular Joint:* The patient is requested to open and close his or her mouth.
> *Shoulder Girdle:* The patient shrugs the shoulders up to the ears and depresses them.
> *Glenohumeral Joint:* The patient moves the arm through elevation (OP).
> *Elbow Joint:* The patient bends the elbow as far as he or she can with the forearm supinated (OP). Next, the patient is asked to straighten the elbow (OP).
> *Radio-ulnar Joint:* The forearm is actively supinated (OP). The forearm is actively pronated (OP).
> *Wrist Joint:* The wrist joint is extended (OP), then flexed (OP).
> *Fingers:* The fingers are actively flexed into the palm of the hand (OP) and then extended (OP).

Muscle Power and Myotomes

To determine the integrity of the nerve roots rising from the different segments, a muscle (or muscles) supplied by an individual nerve root is tested isometrically. (Repeated testing may be necessary before slight weakness is revealed.) Muscle weakness and/or pain is recorded.

Short pivot flexion.	C1
Short pivot extension.	C2
Lateral flexion.	C3 (Figure 4-1)
Shoulder elevators.	C3, 4
Shoulder abductors.	C5
Elbow flexors.	C6 (Figure 4-2)
Elbow extensors.	C7
Wrist extensors.	C6 (C7)
Wrist flexors.	C7
Thumb extensors.	C8
Finger adductors.	T1

Note: Care must be taken when performing isometric tests to ensure that the patient is stabilized adequately. To achieve this, it may be necessary to do some testing with the patient in the supine position. For example, let us suppose that a patient has a painful shoulder problem and during the scan as the myotome for C6 (biceps) is being tested, the shoulder muscles contract strongly to stabilize the shoulder. This strong contraction could produce pain in the shoulder causing the patient to produce an erroneous weak response when the biceps is being tested. By placing the patient in the supine position the shoulder is stabilized, and the therapist is able to reinforce this stabilization with one hand while testing biceps with the other.

Reflexes

The following reflexes can be tested for further evidence of nerve root integrity.

Biceps	C5, C6
Brachioradialis	C6
Triceps	C7

The interpretation of the findings of muscle weakness and pain was described in Chapters 2 and 3.

Sensation

Finally, in the scan examination, it is necessary to test the different dermatomes for evidence of sensory changes.

Note: It is the author's opinion that the scan examination should never be excluded from a musculoskeletal examination. The information obtained facilitates the identification of the area containing the structure at fault. In addition, it provides a valuable data base that can be reinforced with the findings from the detailed examination.

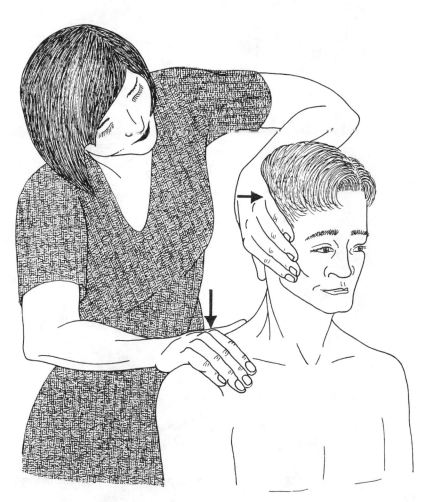

Figure 4-1. Stabilization of the shoulder during the right isometric lateral flexion test for the cervical spine.

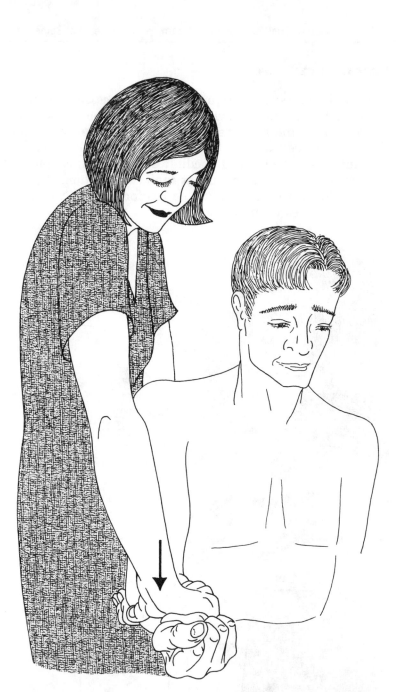

Figure 4-2. Stabilization of the right upper extremity when testing for the C6 myotome.

DETAILED EXAMINATION OF THE CERVICAL SPINE

This section provides a brief review of the essential surface anatomy of the region. The detailed examination section includes a description of Maitland's passive accessory movements and quadrant tests, followed by a discussion of the McKenzie approach.

Surface Anatomy

Surface anatomy involves observing the superficial muscles and bony landmarks of the region being examined.

Posterior view

When examining the cervical spine from a posterior view, do the following:

1. Locate the external occipital protuberance at the upper end of the median furrow at the back of the neck.
2. Take note of the superior nuchal lines (the ridges moving laterally from the occipital protuberance); they are the muscle attachment areas for the posterior capitis muscles.
3. Identify the inion which is the most salient point of the occipital protuberance.
4. The posterior arch of the atlas cannot be felt, but the suboccipital muscles can be located lying deep in this region between the occiput and C2 (palpation is facilitated in the supine position).
5. The spinous process of C2 is a large, biped structure that is easily palpable. It lies on a level with the angle of the jaw.
6. The spinous processes of C3 and C4 are not readily palpable because C2 overhangs them, and they are lost in the normal posterior concavity of the cervical spine. However, with the cervical spine in flexion it is possible to locate them. Failing this they may have to be palpated with the patient in the supine position.
7. The spinous process of C5 is palpable and that of C6 can be recognized easily since it appears to disappear when the cervical spine is extended.

8. There are two more vertebrae that are useful landmarks. The first is T3 which lies on a level with the spine of the scapula. The second is T7 which can be located on the same level as the inferior angle of the scapula.
9. The facet joints, forming the articular pillar, are located one inch from the spinous processes. The inferior articular facets can be palpated through the paravertebral muscles as small bumps. The tips of the spinous processes C2 to C6 lie on a level with the lower margin of the inferior articular facet of the corresponding facet joint, for example, the tip of C5 spinous process lies on a level with the lowest margin of the C5 to C6 facet joint.

Lateral view

When examining the cervical spine from a lateral view, do the following:

1. The joint line of the temporo-mandibular joint can be palpated by placing the tip of the index finger about one centimeter anterior to the tragus of the ear.
2. Locate the mastoid bone which lies behind the ear on a line level with the tragus.
3. The transverse process of C1 can be palpated on a line connecting the mastoid bone with the angle of the jaw. It is a small round button of bone which is tender on pressure.
4. The transverse processes of the remaining cervical vertebrae lie in a convex line just anterior to the anterior border of the sternomastoid.
5. The scalene muscles can be palpated in the posterior triangle of the neck just behind the posterior border of the sternomastoid muscle.

Component Parts of a Typical Vertebra

Figure 4-3 shows the component parts of a typical vertebra (Kapandji, 1974). A typical vertebra consists of the following parts from posterior to anterior.

1. Spinous process
2. The vertebral arch, formed posteriorly by the laminae and anteriorly by the pedicles

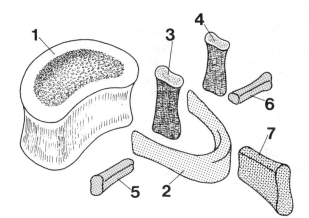

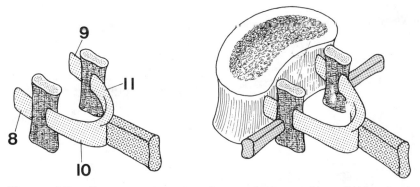

Figure 4-3. Component parts of a typical vertebra. **1.** Vertebral body, **2.** Vertebral arch, **3. & 4.** Articular processes, **5. & 6.** Transverse processes, **7.** Spinous process, **8. & 9.** Pedicles, **10. & 11.** Laminae. (Adapted from Kapandji, 1972).

3. The articular processes and, in close proximity, the transverse processes
4. The most anteriorly situated structure, the vertebral body.

The Functional Unit

This unit (Figure 4-4) is composed of two vertebrae lying one on top of the other with the intervertebral disc between. The functional unit exhibits both static and dynamic qualities. The vertebral body is responsible for the static qualities which are largely weight bearing. The intervertebral disc, the facet joint (which can be regarded as a fulcrum), and the ligamentous complex constitute the dynamic aspects of the functional unit. The ligamentous structures in Figure 4-4 are:

1. Anterior longitudinal ligament
2. Posterior longitudinal ligament
3. Ligamentum flavum
4. Interspinous ligament
5. Ligamentum nuchae.

Movement between one vertebra and another is slight, but the cumulative effect of these movements throughout the cervical spine affords considerable movement.

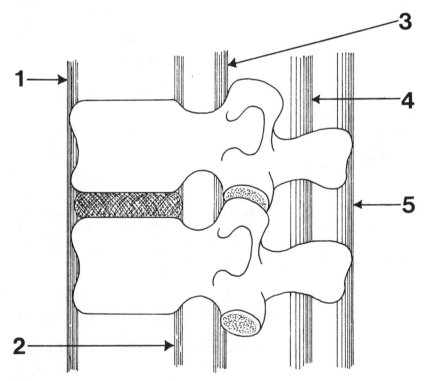

Figure 4-4. Functional unit and ligamentous complex. **1.** Anterior longitudinal ligament, **2.** Posterior longitudinal ligament, **3.** Ligamentum flavum, **4.** Interspinous ligament, **5.** Ligamentum nuchae.

The Intervertebral Foramen

This unit is formed anteriorly by the disc and part of the vertebral body. The capsule of the facet joint and the ligamentum flavum form the posterior border. The roof and the floor are formed from the pedicles of adjacent vertebrae. Contained within the intervertebral foramen are:

- the spinal nerve
- the dural sleeve
- blood vessels
- connective tissue and fat.

Clinically the intervertebral foramen has great significance. Under normal circumstances, there is adequate space within the foramen to accommodate the sensitive nerve root and dural sleeve, even when the size of the foramen is compromised during certain movements of the cervical spine. However, traumatic incidents resulting in herniations of discs, subluxations of the facet joints, or the formation of osteophytes from degenerative processes may compromise the size of the foramen to the extent that the nerve root and the dural sleeve are irritated. When this happens, nerve root syndromes develop.

Nerve Root Syndromes
in the Cervical Spine

The classical signs and symptoms associated with nerve root irritation were described in Chapter 1. However they are worthy of reiteration.

A patient who is suffering from nerve root irritation could present with all or some of the following signs and symptoms.

1. Lancinating shooting pain in the corresponding dermatome, which may or may not be accompanied by distal paresthesia;
2. Muscle weakness in the associated myotome;
3. A sluggish reflex response; and/or
4. Sensory loss in the dermatome.

As stated previously, a patient may not present all of those signs and symptoms. For the diagnosis of nerve root irritation to be made, muscle weakness or paresthesia must be present. Otherwise, the painful symptoms could be the result of somatic reference. Sluggish reflexes can be present in normal individuals.

The following nerve root syndromes occur frequently (Cyriax, 1982).

C5 Nerve Root

Pain in the C5 dermatome
Weakness of deltoid, the spinati, and biceps
Sluggish or absent reflexes in biceps and brachioradialis

C6 Nerve Root

Pain in C6 dermatome
Paresthesia of thumb and index finger
Weakness of extensor carpi radialis, biceps, and brachialis
Sluggish or absent biceps reflex

C7 Nerve Root

Pain in the dermatome
Paresthesia index, long and ring finger
Weakness of triceps, wrist flexors, and latissimus dorsi

C8 Nerve Root

Pain in the dermatome
Paresthesia of long, ring, and little finger
Weakness of extensor pollicis longus, adductor pollicis, flexor carpi ulnaris, and adduction of index finger

Compressing and Stretching Effects of Movements of the Cervical Spine

Grieve (1981) discusses compressing and stretching effects.

Flexion

Posterior structures are stretched and the anterior structures are compressed.
The size of the intervertebral foramen is increased.

Extension

Anterior structures are stretched and the posterior structures are compressed. The size of the intervertebral foramen is decreased.

Side flexion

This is accompanied by rotation to the same side. The structures are compressed on the side to which the head is side flexed and stretched on the opposite side. The size of the intervertebral foramen is decreased on the compressed side.

Rotation

This is accompanied by side flexion to the same side. The size of the intervertebral foramen is decreased on the side to which the head is rotated.

DETAILED EXAMINATION

Resisted isometric contractions, which are an essential feature of the detailed examination of the peripheral joints and the upper quadrant screening examination, are not repeated in the detailed examination of the cervical spine. There are two reasons for this. First, except in exceptional circumstances (e.g., trauma), the muscular components of the cervical spine are not affected in the same way as they are in the peripheral joints. However, muscle tightness, spasm, and imbalance of the muscles of the cervical spine can have significant ramifications extending beyond the cervical spine (Yanda, 1988). Second, the structure of the cervical spine, composed as it is of segments, makes it difficult to obtain a pure isometric response.

Passive Intervertebral Movements

Figure 4-5 illustrates the application of direct pressures to parts of the vertebra (Maitland, 1986). The purpose of performing these movements is to confirm the segment containing the lesion at fault by eliciting the signs and symptoms of which the patient is complaining.

- *Procedure:* These procedures are performed with the patient in the prone position with the forehead supported on the backs of the hands and the thorax supported on a pillow. The therapist stands at the end of the plinth nearest the patient's head, and applies gentle pressures in a posteroanterior (P-A) direction on the spinous processes with the tips of the thumbs (Figure 4-5a). The gentle pressures are transmitted from the shoulders down the arms through the thumbs, which are placed together with the nails facing each other; the fingers remain relaxed at either side of the patient's neck. The P-A movements may be repeated over the articular pillars if necessary (Figure 4-5b). Finally transverse pressures can be applied to the lateral surface of the spinous processes (Figure 4-5c).

Specific Tests

Sometimes the scan examination does not implicate the cervical spine as being the area containing the lesion. Yet the therapist may feel, after taking the patient's history, that the cervical spine is the culprit. Under these circumstances, certain tests can be performed to elicit cervical symptoms.

Compression Test and Distraction Test

This test, as its name suggests, adds further compression to the cervical structures on the side which is thought to be affected.

- *Procedure.* With the patient in the sitting position and the head extended and rotated to the affected side, the examiner places his or her clasped hands on top of the patient's head and applies a downward pressure. Reproduction of the patient's symptoms confirms that the cervical spine contains the lesion. Conversely, distraction of the cervical spine is used as a test to determine whether relief of symptoms will be achieved.

Maitland's Cervical Quadrant Tests

These two tests combine movements to produce maximum compression on one side of the cervical spine and maximum stretch on the other. Symptoms may be elicited from either the compression or the stretch.

Upper Cervical Quadrant Test. This is a combination of passive upper cervical extension, with rotation and lateral flexion to the same side.

Lower Cervical Quadrant Test. The lower cervical region is passively extended, side flexed, and rotated to the same side.

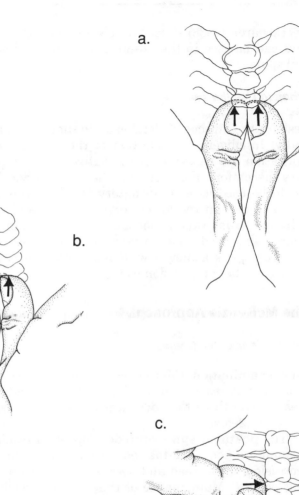

Figure 4-5. Application of direct pressures to parts of the vertebra: (a) posteroanterior pressures on the spinous process, (b) posteroanterior unilateral vertebral pressures on the articular pillar, and (c) transverse pressures on the lateral surface of the spinous process. (Adapted from Maitland, 1986).

Edwards (1988) describes a series of combined movements that can be used in the examination and treatment of the cervical spine.

When to Use the Tests

Tests in the musculoskeletal examination are not used automatically. Intelligence in selection of the test and prudence in its utilization are necessary if the patient is to be spared unnecessary discomfort. For instance, the lower cervical quadrant test would be used as a confirmatory test if it were thought that a lesion existed in the lower cervical spine, and the information achieved so far was inconclusive. Utilization of this test would negate the need to do the compression test, because more compression is achieved with the lower cervical quadrant test than with the compression test.

The McKenzie Approach

The McKenzie Syndromes

This examination (McKenzie, 1990) is based on three syndromes that respond to testing and treatment by mechanical means. The three disorders are those of posture, dysfunction, and derangement.

The **postural syndrome** develops as a result of the patient assuming a poor, habitual posture. In the cervical spine, this is protrusion of the head and neck accompanied by a slouched sitting posture. Maintenance of this position inevitably results in pain, and it is only by correcting the position that the pain is relieved. As might be expected, the pain is intermittent, only developing on assumption of prolonged postures.

The **dysfunction syndrome**, as its name suggests, develops as a result of a patient avoiding certain full-range movements of the cervical spine. Contractures develop in the soft tissues, and the patient experiences pain when those structures are subjected to stretch at the end of range. The syndrome may develop over time as a result of habitual poor posture or may be the aftermath of a derangement or trauma. The pain is intermittent. During the assessment process, the painful end range of movement is detected and that movement is used to remodel the collagen fibers by encouraging the patient to gently stretch the contracted structures.

A **derangement** is considered to be due to the displacement of nuclear material toward the periphery of the disc and beyond. Unlike the other syndromes, the pain in a derangement syndrome is often constant and can change location. The pain develops as a result of interference in the normal flow of the fluid nucleus and the adverse effect on movements of the cervical spine.

The symptoms from a derangement can be local in nature in that they are experienced close to the spinal column, or they can radiate into the extremity in the form of pain, numbness, or paresthesia. When pain, felt locally, begins to radiate down into the upper extremity, the term **peripheralization** is used. When pain in the extremity begins to recede and becomes localized in the cervical spine, the term **centralization** is used. The object in the assessment process is to determine which movements cause centralization of pain, or reduction of the patient's pain, and to use those movements in the treatment process.

Some Aspects of The McKenzie Examination of the Cervical Spine

The following is the author's interpretation of the McKenzie examination of the cervical spine (McKenzie, 1990) which consists of three parts.

1. *Exercises to Determine the Quality of Movement.* Each exercise is performed once only, but maximum available range within the patient's pain tolerance must be achieved. As each exercise is performed, the quality of the movement (ease of performance, pure movement without deviation, and so on) is recorded. Range of motion is recorded in terms of the restriction noted, for example, major, moderate, or minor. The exercises are: flexion, extension, rotation, and lateral flexion.

2. *Dynamic Test Movements.* These exercises are performed 5 to 15 times each and a notation is made of the effect of the exercise on the patient's pain. Does it make it better? Does it make it worse? Is there any change? In terms of making the pain better in the presence of a derangement, centralization is the aim, whereas peripheralization would indicate a worsening of the patient's pain. Following are descriptions of the exercises.

• *Head protrusion in sitting.* The patient is in the sitting position in a high backed chair. From the neutral position, the patient is encouraged to stretch the neck forward as far as possible, maintaining a horizontal gaze without either an upward or downward movement, occurring. On completion of this movement, it will be noted that the upper cervical spine is extended and the lower is flexed.

• *Head retraction in sitting.* This is the reverse of the previous exercise. The patient is instructed to pull the chin in as far as possible in a horizontal direction. Again, upward or downward movement should be avoided. The exercise is not easy to perform in terms of achieving maximum range, and the patient may require further instruction in the technique.

Head retraction with overpressure from the patient's fingers on the chin should be introduced if the previous exercise has had no effect on the patient's pain.

• *Retraction and extension in sitting.* Head retraction as just described is performed first, and then the patient extends the head and neck cautiously and slowly over the back of the chair achieving as much extension as pain will permit. The performance of head retraction prior to extension achieves more extension in the lower cervical spine than does extension alone.

If there is no change in the patient's pain when this exercise is repeated 5 to 15 times, rotation is introduced at the limit of the patient's available range of extension. The rotary component is achieved by instructing the patient to move the nose half an inch to the right, then to the left of mid-line. The addition of the rotary component enables the patient to move further into extension in a relaxed manner, and since the weight of the head constitutes overpressure a maximum range is achieved.

If the patient cannot perform this exercise in the sitting position, it can be performed in the supine position with the patient's head, neck, and shoulders clear of the edge of the plinth. The patient supports the head with the hand and lowers the head and neck slowly into extension until full extension is achieved, and the head and neck are in the relaxed hanging position.

• *Lateral flexion in sitting.* The patient is instructed to retract the head and then to side flex to the painful side maintaining the laterally flexed position for a second or so. The patient then returns the head to the neutral position. The exercise is repeated 5 to 15 times.

If that exercise has no effect on the patient's pain the following progression is introduced. The patient stabilizes the trunk by gripping the seat of the chair with the hand on the nonpainful side. He or she then places the hand of the affected side over the top of the head so that the finger tips overlap the ear on the nonpainful side and, with the head retracted, pulls the head into lateral flexion. This produces a passive overpressure.

• *Rotation.* The patient is again in the sitting position with the head retracted. He or she is encouraged to rotate the head toward the side of pain, hold for a second, and return to the neutral position. The exercise is repeated 5 to 15 times.

If there is no change in the patient's symptoms, the patient can provide overpressure by placing the hand of the affected side under the chin, with the other hand embracing the occiput and lateral part of the head. He or she then moves the retracted head into rotation to the painful side.

• *Flexion.* With the patient in the slouched sitting position, so that the spine is flexed, the patient is encouraged to bend the head forward so that the chin rests on the chest. He or she then returns the head to the neutral position and the exercise is repeated 5 to 15 times.

Once again, in the event that there is no change in the patient's symptoms, the patient can apply overpressure. He or she does this by clasping the hands behind the back of the head and bringing the head down to rest on the chest.

3. *Static Mechanical Postural Testing.* Although the exercises just described can be used to determine the presence of a derangement or dysfunction, they would be ineffective in terms of detecting a postural problem. However, with some modification they can be used to determine whether the patient's problem is due to a poor posture of the head and neck. The modification involves utilizing the following exercises, but instead of moving quickly into them and out of them as was done with the dynamic tests, the position is maintained at the end of range for about 3 minutes. This should provide sufficient time to reproduce the patient's symptoms. Normally the postures need only be assumed once, but again the end of range must be achieved. The positions assumed are as follows.

• head protrusion with the patient in the sitting slouched position;

• head retraction with the patient in sitting;
• lying supine in extension with head retraction; and
• lying prone in extension.

The last exercise in the above list has not been mentioned before and will be described now. The patient is in the prone position leaning on his or her elbows. The outstretched finger tips are beneath the chin so that the head is facing forward and upward. The position is maintained for 3 minutes.

SUMMARY

In this chapter, the upper quadrant screening examination was described in detail and included observation for postural discrepancies, tests for peripheral joints, myotomes, nerve root integrity, and sensory testing of dermatomes and reflexes. Of particular importance were the tests described to determine the cause of dizziness. Surface anatomy provided the means of identifying important structures of the cervical spine by palpation prior to performing the detailed examination. The functional unit and the clinically important intervertebral foramen were described. Passive intervertebral movements were utilized to determine the segment at fault, special tests were utilized eclectically to confirm earlier findings. Finally, an interpretation of part of the Mckenzie assessment of the cervical spine was discussed.

CHAPTER 5

• • • • • • • •

The Shoulder Complex

The shoulder complex is vulnerable to injury. This is particularly so of the glenohumeral joint which is designed for mobility rather than stability. It is subject to repetitive strain injuries, traumatic injuries and those of a degenerative nature. The movement of the component parts of the complex are integrated; consequently, a problem affecting one joint could affect the others.

The shoulder complex consists of the following joints: the scapulothoracic physiological joint; the acromioclavicular joint; the sternoclavicular joint; the glenohumeral joint; and the subdeltoid physiological joint (Figure 5-1). The articular surfaces of this joint are the head of the humerus, covered by the rotator cuff muscles, and the subdeltoid bursa (Kapandji, 1982).

The function of these joints is to facilitate movement of the upper extremity to ensure appropriate placing of the hand for effective use. The joints are interdependent and move in concert with one another. The movements of the upper extremity determine the varying contribution made by the different joints. Kapandji (1982) describes direct links between the first three joints listed and direct links between the last two joints. It follows then that a problem with one of these joints could affect the function of the others.

Cailliet (1988) and Kaput (1987) both feel that the costosternal and costovertebral joints should be included when

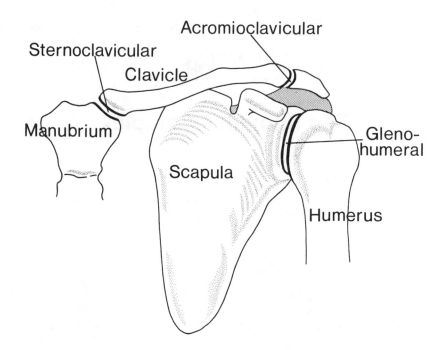

Figure 5-1. The major joints in the shoulder girdle complex and associated bony structures.

describing the shoulder complex. Although it is important to bear these joints in mind, they are not generally included in an assessment of the shoulder complex.

Wells (1982) has pointed out that painful disorders of the glenohumeral joint frequently have their origin in the cervical spine. Maigne (1972) believes that an examination of the cervical spine should be carried out wherever a painful shoulder exists. Kessel (1982) has stated that in one fifth of patients with shoulder pain, the pain is referred from the cervical spine. Indeed, clearance of the cervical spine is an important preliminary step in solving problems involving the shoulder complex.

By far the most common afflictions of the shoulder complex are those involving the soft tissue structures of the glenohumeral joint. Neer (1983) has identified the supraspinatus, and the biceps tendon as the most common structures involved.

Certainly these tendons are prone to overuse syndromes. The supraspinatus is particularly vulnerable.

Problems involving the acromioclavicular joint are fairly common in athletes; these problems usually result in a partial or complete separation of the joint. Other problems, involving a strain or sprain of the joint, can develop from overuse as a result of abnormal mobility elsewhere in the complex, for example, the scapulothoracic mechanism.

SURFACE ANATOMY

The location of significant bony landmarks and soft tissue structures are described below.

Acromion

If the spine of the scapula is followed to its lateral end, the fingers will come into contact with a bony shelf overlying the head of the humerus. This is the acromion process.

Head of the Humerus

If the pad of the index finger is allowed to slide laterally off the shelf-like acromion, it will come to lie on the lateral aspect of the head of the humerus. The anterosuperior aspect can be palpated by moving the index finger in an anterior direction.

Greater Tuberosity

This is the prominence that can be palpated beneath the deltoid. It and the bulk of deltoid do, in fact, provide the shoulder with its rounded contour. Its lateral and anterior borders can be palpated.

Lesser Tuberosity

Once the greater tuberosity has been located, the lesser tuberosity can be palpated by moving anteromedially in a straight line.

Coracoid Process

This lies about one inch below the concavity in the lateral one third of the clavicle.

SOFT TISSUE STRUCTURES

The following soft tissue structures are the most vulmerable in terms of developing tendonitis. The first two are thought to have areas of avascularity and, as stated earlier, they are prone to overuse syndromes.

Long Head of Biceps

This lies in the groove between the two tuberosities. It is a round tendon that is easier to palpate with the elbow bent and the shoulder externally rotated.

Supraspinatus Tendon

This can be revealed by asking the patient to place the hand behind the back, thus bringing the upper part of the humerus forward from beneath the acromion; the supraspinatus is the flat structure lying just below the anterior edge of the acromion.

Infraspinatus Tendon

This tendon lies just behind that of supraspinatus on the greater tuberosity. It is easy to palpate if the patient is in the forearm support prone position with the elbow lying directly beneath the shoulder and slightly adducted. The patient's hand grips the edge of the plinth. The tendon can be palpated just below the lateral end of the spine of the scapula.

DETAILED EXAMINATION

The screening examination (the Upper Quadrant scan) will have been performed and the cervical spine cleared (see previous chapters). The scan will have revealed the area(s) containing the lesion at fault and details from the patient's medical history such as:

- location of pain
- description of the pain — burning, stabbing, constant, intermittent
- severity — scale of 1 to 10
- irritability — type of activity that increases the pain; severity of increased symptoms; length of time the increased symptoms last
- abnormalities of sensation
- loss or change in functional ability in daily activities or occupation.

During observation, postural abnormalities, abrasions, bruising, changes in bony and soft tissue contours such as atrophy, and so on, would have been noted.

The detailed examination of the joints of the shoulder complex will be described next. The examination is described for the patient's **right** side.

The Scapulothoracic Mechanism

The scapulohumeral rhythm depends on the relationship between the glenohumeral movement and the movement of the scapula on the posterior chest wall. Under normal circumstances, this ratio is approximately 2:1. Thus, if there are 180° of motion during elevation through abduction, then the movement of the scapula should be responsible for 60°. A "reversed" scapulohumeral rhythm is said to exist if there is restriction of motion in the glenohumeral joint, and the scapula becomes hypermobile in an attempt to counteract this restriction.

Of particular interest in terms of observation is the position of the scapula on the posterior chest wall. Under normal circumstances, the glenoid fossa is directed anteriorly, upward and laterally. Any deviations in the normal position of the scapula will change the orientation of the glenoid and so affect the stable base required for movements of the upper limb (Peat, 1986).

Mobilization of the Scapula

The movements for mobilization of the scapula are elevation, depression, retraction (adduction), and protraction (abduction), and medial (downward) and lateral (upward) rotation (Figure 5-2).

- *Position of patient:* The patient is in the left-side lying position facing the examiner.
- *Grips:* The therapist's proximal grip lies on the superior aspect of the shoulder girdle with the fingers overlapping the spine of the scapula and pointing in a caudal direction. The distal grip embraces the inferior angle with the fingers lying in contact with the medial border and the thumb lying against the lateral border.
- *Procedure:* The therapist passively moves the scapula into **elevation** with the distal grip, at the same time as the weight is transferred onto the right foot. The proximal grip remains relaxed. **Depression** is achieved by transferring the body weight from the right foot to the left at the same time as the fingers of the proximal grip gently move the spine of the scapula in a caudal direction, while the distal grip remains relaxed. The end feel is noted — soft tissue resistance.

   It is important to detect early signs of resistance (R1) and the final resistance to motion (R2) in all the following movements.

   With the hands in the same position, the therapist can test **retraction** by applying a medial thrust with the thumb of the distal grip and a medial glide with the fingers of the proximal grip, at the same time as the weight is transferred onto the forward foot. **Protraction** is achieved by relaxing the thumb and using the fingers of the distal grip to glide the scapula toward the therapist, assisted by the fingers of the proximal grip. The weight is transferred to the back foot. Again the end feel is noted.

   Medial and lateral rotation are tested, again utilizing the same grips; the therapist swivels his or her right hip posteriorly to test medial rotation and anteriorly to test lateral rotation.

Scapular Lift

The patient is in the prone position with the right hand placed behind his or her back. The therapist's right hand, placed anteriorly on the shoulder, eases the shoulder girdle into some retraction at the same time that the therapist's left hand lifts

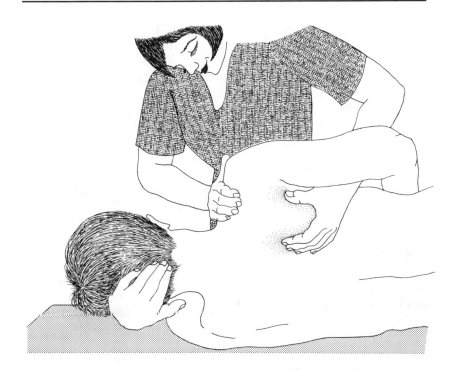

Figure 5-2. Mobilization of the scapula.

up the medial border of the scapula by curling the fingers underneath.

If the passive movements of the scapula are full and pain free, the strength of the muscles controlling the scapula can be determined by having the patient actively perform the scapula movements isometrically against the resistance applied by the therapist.

The Acromioclavicular (AC) and the Sternoclavicular (SC) Joints

The accessory movements that take place at these joints are those of elevation and depression and anterior and posterior glides. Elevation makes a significant contribution to abduction of the glenohumeral joint beyond 100°. The anterior and pos-

terior gliding mechanisms are essential to the smooth performance of flexion and extension at the glenohumeral joint (Peat,
1986).

These movements can be tested by having the patient in the
supine position and simply picking up the lateral clavicle with
the right hand and moving it in a superior and inferior direction and then in an anterior and posterior direction (Mennell,
1964). The index finger of the therapist's left hand detects
movement in the AC joint as the clavicle is moved, and this is
compared with the opposite side.

Alternatively, movements at the AC joint can be tested with
the patient in a sitting position; the therapist's right hand
provides support around the glenohumeral joint, with the index
finger stabilizing the acromion anteriorly; the left thumb and
index finger perform the anterior and posterior gliding movements on the lateral clavicle (Figure 5-3). Similarly, the
sternoclavicular joint can be tested with the patient in the
supine position for anterior and posterior glides and for
elevation and depression (Figure 5-4).

The Glenohumeral Joint

The close packed position for this joint is abduction and lateral
rotation; the loose packed position is semiabduction. The
testing movements for the glenohumeral joint can be performed
with the patient in the sitting or lying position. The choice
depends on the most comfortable position for the patient and
the utilization of good body mechanics by the therapist.

Although disorders of this joint can usually be detected by
utilizing 12 movements (Cyriax, 1982), an active hand behind
the head followed by a hand behind the back will provide the
therapist with valuable initial information.

The Testing Movements

The following movements will stress the contractile and inert
structures associated with the glenohumeral joint. In the
presence of pathology, they will elicit signs or symptoms.

Active Elevation Through Abduction Since this is an active
movement, it does not tell the therapist anything definite. It
indicates the patient's willingness to move, gives some indica-

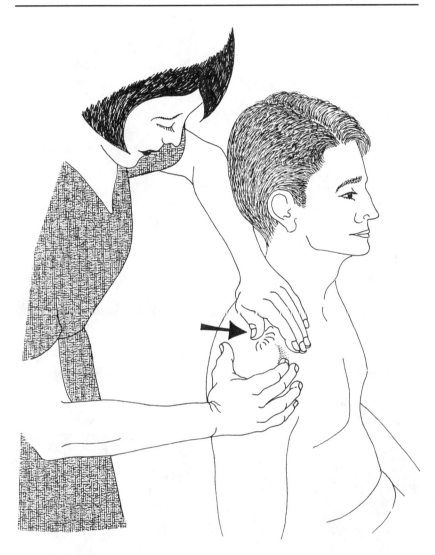

Figure 5-3. Anterior glide of the lateral clavicle.

tion of available range of motion, and whether that range is pain free. It also provides the therapist with the opportunity to observe the scapulohumeral rhythm. Finally, the presence of a painful arc may be detected.

Passive Elevation Through Abduction For the performance of this movement, the therapist asks the patient to relax the arm

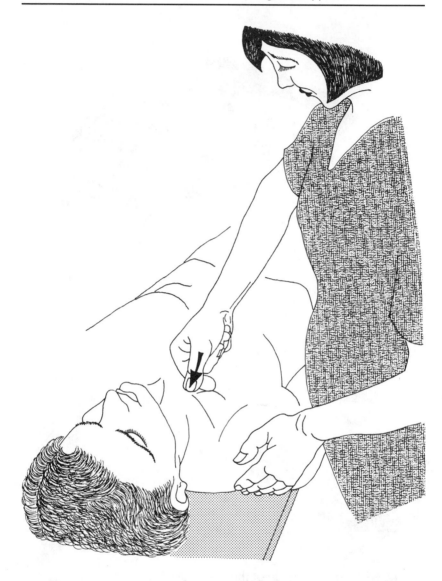

Figure 5-4. Posterior glide of the medial clavicle.

while the therapist passively moves it through the available range of motion. The end feel is noted and should feel free rather than exhibit the characteristic hard end feel of capsular restriction. Pain experienced long before end of range is reached with a soft end feel is indicative of a subdeltoid bursitis. Pain experienced at extremes of motion, but in the absence of a capsular end feel, implicates a chronic condition, for example, bursitis, tendonitis, or acromioclavicular joint problem. With any of these conditions, overpressure will increase the pain.

Passive Abduction To test this movement, the therapist must fix the scapula by exerting a medial force against the lateral border of the scapula with the thumb and thenar eminence, or by placing the left hand on the shoulder girdle and fixing it as the shoulder is abducted. Limitation here could indicate that a capsular pattern is present. Pain at the extreme of the range could be due to a strain of the acromioclavicular joint.

Passive Lateral Rotation This movement is performed with the arm at the side and the elbow flexed to 90°. The therapist passively rotates the arm in a lateral direction. Painful restriction may be due to a capsular pattern; a pain free restriction demonstrated bilaterally could be due to normal loss of range as part of the aging process. Pain at the extreme of motion could again mean there is a strain of the acromioclavicular joint.

Passive Medial Rotation Kessel (1982) suggests that this movement be performed with the arms at the sides, and the elbows straight. Marked epicondyles provide reference points for comparing the affected side with the sound side. If the movement is performed with the arm in the same position as for lateral rotation, the forearm will come into contact with the body before full range is reached.

Painful restriction of motion could mean that the capsular pattern is present. The acromioclavicular joint is implicated if pain is experienced at the extreme of motion. Sometimes a painful arc is present, indicating that a painful structure is being impinged on.

Passive Horizontal Adduction With his or her right arm, the therapist supports the patient's arm, which is bent at the elbow, while the therapist's left hand stabilizes the patient's left scapular region. The patient's arm is then moved horizontally across the chest. This is the classical test for the acromioclavicular joint.

For the following **resisted isometric contractions**, the therapist is trying to achieve a strong contraction of the muscle(s) being tested. This is done by slowly building up a resistance and getting the patient to hold the position while matching the therapist's resistance. Care must be taken to avoid any isotonic activity or a false result will be obtained. Counter pressure is applied with the therapist's other hand. The therapist is trying to elicit weakness or pain, or a combination of both. Weakness can be due to lack of use, a nerve root problem, or other neuropathy. A painful result is due to involvement of a contractile structure, that is, a tendon, muscle belly, and so on.

Resisted Abduction Clinically, it has been found that if this contraction produces pain it is due to supraspinatus tendonitis. Theoretically, of course, it could be due to deltoid strain, but this muscle is rarely affected.

Resisted Adduction A painful response to this test is probably due to a strain of one of the adductor muscles.

Resisted Lateral Rotation Pain produced here is most likely due to infraspinatus tendonitis rather than teres minor involvement.

Resisted Medial Rotation Subscapularis tendonitis (rare) could be the causative factor if a painful response is produced; the other possibility is adductor strain.

Resisted Elbow Flexion Although any of the elbow flexors could be involved with a painful response to this test, usually biceps is the culprit. Special tests will confirm this.

Resisted Elbow Extension This movement rarely produces a painful response; a weak response implicates the nerve supply to triceps.

The Accessory Movements

The following list outlines the accessory movements and the physiological movements with which they are associated.

- lateral distraction (Kaltenborn, 1989) as a means of separating the joint surfaces, and for general mobilization
- inferior glide (associated with abduction)
- anterior glide (associated with extension, external rotation, and horizontal abduction)
- posterior glide (associated with flexion, internal rotation, and horizontal adduction)

Note: The following procedures are only necessary if restriction of joint motion has been detected in the physiological movements. If no restriction has been detected, the following assessment procedures can be eliminated.

Testing General Mobility

To assess the general mobility of the patient before beginning accessory movements, do the following:

- *Position of the patient:* The patient is supine with the right arm in the resting position.
- *Position of the therapist:* The therapist stands level with the patient's right shoulder.
- *Grips:* The therapist's hands embrace the head of the humerus. The web between the thumb and index finger of the therapist's left hand embraces the superior aspect of the head of the humerus so that the index finger lies posteriorly and the thumb anteriorly. The patient's shoulder is supported in approximately 55° of abduction and 30° of flexion. The therapist's right forearm supports the patient's forearm near the wrist.
- *Procedure:* By adjusting the thrust through the hands, the therapist can test the mobility of the humeral head in an anterior, posterior, superior, and inferior direction.

Lateral Distraction

Figure 5-5 illustrates the procedure to follow for lateral distraction.

- *Position of the patient:* The patient is in the supine position with the shoulder in the resting position and the elbow flexed.
- *Position of the therapist:* The therapist stands facing the patient.

- *Proximal grip:* This is placed on the medial aspect of the upper end of the humerus close to the axilla.
- *Distal grip:* The therapist's left hand is placed just above the elbow on the lateral side and provides gentle support.
- *Procedure:* The therapist takes up the slack with the proximal grip and then thrusts the upper end of the humerus in a lateral direction until distraction of the joint is achieved.

Note: The alternative approach is for the therapist to use a belt which goes around the upper end of the humerus and then around the therapist's waist. Distraction is achieved by the therapist leaning backward.

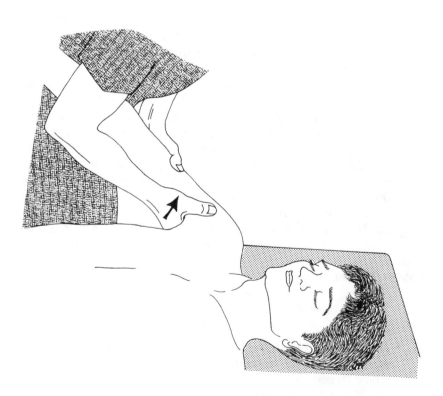

Figure 5-5. Lateral distraction of the head of the humerus.

Inferior Glide

Figure 5-6 illustrates the inferior glide movement.

- *Position of the patient:* The patient is supine with the right arm in the resting position.
- *Position of the therapist:* The therapist stands level with the patient's right shoulder.
- *Proximal grip:* The therapist's hands embrace the head of the humerus. The web between the thumb and index finger of the therapist's left hand embraces the superior aspect of the humerus so that the fingers lie posteriorly and the thumb anteriorly on the head of the humerus.
- *Distal grip:* The web space between the index finger and the thumb of the therapist's right hand lies loosely in contact with the inferior aspect of the head of the humerus; the thumb is placed anteriorly and the rest of the fingers posteriorly on the head of the humerus.
- *Procedure:* The therapist thrusts down with the web space of the left hand and displaces the head of the humerus inferiorly.

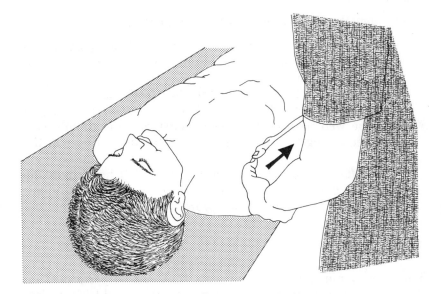

Figure 5-6. Inferior glide of the head of the humerus.

Anterior Glide

The anterior glide procedure is accomplished by doing the following:

- *Position of the patient:* For all of the following procedures, the patient is in the sitting position with the arm in about 55° of abduction and 30° of flexion.
- *Position of the therapist:* For all of the following procedures, the therapist is sitting facing the patient's arm with the patient's shoulder at the level of the therapist's chest.
- *Proximal grip:* The therapist's right hand fixes the shoulder girdle with the index finger placed against the acromion and the thumb in the axilla. The patient's wrist is supported by the therapist's forearm.
- *Distal grip:* The therapist's left hand is placed against the posterior aspect of the head of the humerus so that the web between the thumb and the index finger lies adjacent to the lateral border of the acromion. The thumb lies on top of the head of the humerus with the fingers lying posterior to it.
- *Procedure:* The therapist's left hand glides the head of the humerus forward while the right hand stabilizes the shoulder girdle.

Posterior Glide

To complete the posterior glide procedure, do the following:

- *Proximal grip:* The therapist's left hand lies posterior to the shoulder girdle with the thumb and fingers placed on top of the girdle.
- *Distal grip:* The thumb of the therapist's right hand lies close to the acromion. The head of the humerus is embraced by the web between the index finger and the thumb with the remaining fingers lying beneath the index finger in the axilla.
- *Procedure:* The palm of the therapist's left hand fixes the scapula posteriorly while the therapist's right hand glides the head of the humerus backward.

Special Tests

There are a number of special tests that can be performed on the soft tissue structures associated with the shoulder complex. These are described in the following paragraphs.

Rotator Cuff Mechanism

Partial Tear of the Rotator Cuff (The Drop Arm Test) The patient is instructed to abduct the arm to 90°, then the therapist applies gentle pressure. If the patient is unable to hold the arm in abduction against the gentle pressure of the therapist, a tear of the rotator cuff must be suspected (Hoppenfeld, 1976). Alternatively, having abducted the arm to 90°, the patient is unable to lower it slowly when requested to do so, or may be able to do so but with severe pain (Magee, 1987).

Complete Tear of the Rotator Cuff (The Shoulder Shrug Test) The patient is asked to abduct the arm but is unable to do so and instead shrugs the shoulder. This demonstrates the inability of the rotator cuff muscles to hold the head of the humerus in the glenoid cavity and is indicative of a complete tear of the rotator cuff.

Supraspinatus Tendonitis (The Impingement Sign) The therapist forces the forward flexed arm of the patient against the antero-inferior surface of the acromion. In so doing, the supraspinatus is jammed against the acromion. A positive result is achieved if pain is produced with this maneuver (Hawkins & Abrams, 1987).

An alternative test involves having the patient flex the arm to 90° upon which the therapist internally rotates the arm thus forcing the inflamed part of the tendon against the coraco-acromial ligament. If the patient exhibits a painful response, the test is positive. Hawkins & Abrams (1987) and Neviaser (1987) have indicated that the biceps tendon can also be involved in this test because of its close proximity to the supraspinatus tendon. A differential test for this muscle tendon is described below.

The Long Head of Biceps

Tendonitis of the Long Head of Biceps (Speed's Test) The patient extends the elbow and supinates the forearm then forward flexes the arm against the resistance of the therapist. In the presence of bicipital tendonitis, a painful response will be elicited.

Note: Tendon palpation may add a confirmatory finding.

Shoulder Instabilities

Anterior Instability (The Apprehension Test) The patient's arm is abducted to 90° and then placed slowly and gently into lateral rotation. If instability is present, the patient will demonstrate obvious signs of apprehension and will tend to resist the movement.

Posterior Instability The therapist places the patient's arm in forward flexion to 90°, and in adduction, and then internally rotates the arm in this position. Posterior pressure is applied on the tip of the elbow (Schwartz, Warren, O'Brien, & Fronek, 1987). Once again the patient will demonstrate apprehension and will oppose the movement in the presence of instability.

Schwartz, Warren, O'Brien & Fronek (1987) state that this combination of movements, except for the posterior pressure, is used by the patient to demonstrate voluntary posterior subluxation.

The Upper Limb Tension Test

The upper limb tension test (ULTT) (Kenneally, Rubenach, & Elvey, 1988) was developed by Elvey (1979) in an attempt to differentiate between the cervical spine and the glenohumeral joint as the cause of the patient's shoulder problem. Pain is often referred from the cervical spine to the shoulder; in fact, shoulder pain may be the only pain of which the patient complains. If, under these circumstances, the shoulder is treated and not the neck, the patient's symptoms will not improve. It is known that structures at the site of referred pain can develop secondary pathological changes, such as restriction of movement and pain, that can mask the fact that the cervical spine is the culprit. The longer the shoulder pathology has been in existence the more difficult it is to bring about a reversal of symptoms by treating the cervical spine alone, and it becomes necessary to treat both areas.

Pathological changes in the cervical spine invariably lead to adhesions and fibrous tissue formation around the nerve roots. If this happens the mobility of the nerve roots is restricted, and they become more susceptible to tensile stresses. During the performance of the Elvey test, the nerve roots of the brachial plexus (particularly the upper nerve roots) are put on stretch, and in the presence of cervical spine pathology the patient's pain will be produced.

To avoid stretching structures other than the nerve root (muscles, and so on), the component movements of the test are taken to the end of the pain free range only. For example, if shoulder pain appears or increases when the elbow is extended fully, then the elbow is moved into a pain free range of extension since the pain is probably due to stress on a soft tissue structure other than the nerve root. At the stage of adding the final component, that is, wrist and finger extension, the limb should be pain free. The addition of the last component puts maximum stretch on the upper nerve roots, and if the cervical spine is responsible for the patient's shoulder pain, that pain will be reproduced.

The patient should be warned that he or she may feel a stretch across the joint structures as the different joints in the upper extremity are brought into play.

The test is not infallible, and a positive result is dependent on there being the type of pathology present in the cervical spine that compromises the nerve roots. Consequently, it is possible to have a problem in the cervical spine that is causing the shoulder pain, but which will not result in a positive ULTT.

Finally, the technique described is the basic technique. Sensitivity to the test can be increased by placing the contralateral arm in abduction and lateral rotation or the cervical spine in almost any pain free position before the ULTT is applied. Side flexion of the cervical spine to the contralateral side is commonly used.

Stages and Technique of the ULTT The test is performed in three component parts, and as each part is performed the patient's pain is assessed. The three component parts are:

1. Abduction, extension, and lateral rotation of the shoulder;
2. Full supination followed by extension of the elbow; and
3. Wrist and finger extension.

The test is described for the right side.

- *Position of the patient:* The patient lies in the supine position with the side to be tested close to the edge of the plinth.
- *Position of the therapist:* The therapist half sits on the plinth at the side of the patient close to the right shoulder and facing the patient.

- *Grip:* The therapist's right hand embraces the top of the shoulder girdle with the fingers curling beneath the posterior aspect.
- *Procedure: Movement 1.* With the left hand, the therapist abducts the arm to approximately 110°, or to where maximum tension is exerted since this is going to vary from patient to patient. (The therapist is careful to maintain the mid-range position to avoid any unnecessary stretch on the structures of the shoulder.) The arm is then extended to about 10° beyond the coronal plane (the anterior capsule of the shoulder should not be stressed) and laterally rotated to approximately 60°. The position should be comfortable for the patient and, therefore, movements should not be pushed to the limit. The patient is questioned about any shoulder pain.

    Movement 2: The therapist supinates the arm and slowly extends the elbow. The patient's arm is supported by the therapist's thigh just proximal to the elbow. Once again the patient is questioned regarding shoulder pain.

    Movement 3: If the patient is still not complaining of shoulder pain, then the wrist and fingers are extended. The therapist's right hand moves down to support the elbow as the left hand gently extends the wrist and fingers.

    When Movement 3 has been performed there is maximum stretch on the peripheral nerve or nerve roots. Again the patient is asked about shoulder pain. If the pain has not been reproduced, then the test can be repeated with the addition of one of the sensitizing movements previously mentioned, for example, side flexion of the cervical spine to the left.

As mentioned previously, there are certain stretch responses that are quite normal and must be expected. The patient will experience a stretch across the anterior aspect of the shoulder, a deep stretch sensation across the anterior aspect of the elbow, and tingling in the C6 and C7 dermatomes in the hand. Only if the patient's shoulder pain is reproduced is the ULTT positive.

SUMMARY

In this chapter, bony landmarks were identified and soft tissue structures described. Examination of the scapulothoracic mechanism, the acromioclavicular, sternoclavicular, and glenohumeral joints was discussed as well as the special tests related to the shoulder complex.

CHAPTER 6

• • • • • • • •

The Elbow Complex

There are four joints involved in the elbow complex. The humeroulnar and the humeroradial joints are involved in flexion and extension, and the superior and inferior radioulnar joints participate in pronation and supination.

SURFACE ANATOMY

Cardinal Signs of the Elbow Joint

Under normal circumstances when the elbow is viewed from the posterior aspect with the elbow extended, the two epicondyles and the olecranon process form a straight line. With the elbow flexed, these three bony structures form an isosceles triangle. Deviation from the norm is indicative of new or old fractures in the region.

The Olecranon

This bony prominence is associated with the olecranon bursa which, under normal circumstances, is not palpable. However, it can become quite swollen, particularly in certain arthritic conditions; in this case, it will appear as a distention in the region of the olecranon. The swelling may or may not be painful.

The Epicondyles

These prominences are located as the most lateral and medial projections of the humerus at the elbow. Tenderness of the lateral epicondyle is not an uncommon clinical feature. The most common cause of pain is lateral epicondylitis ("tennis elbow") involving the common extensor tendon muscles. The epicondyle should be palpated on its anterior aspect since this is the most common painful location.

Similarly, the medial epicondyle can give rise to medial epicondylitis associated with a tendonitis of the common flexor tendon. This is commonly known as "golfer's elbow." It is not as severe as lateral epicondylitis or as common.

The Radial Head

This can be palpated just below the lateral epicondyle. Swelling in this region accompanied by pain and restriction in pronation and supination would lead a therapist to suspect the presence of a radial head fracture.

The Cubital Fossa

This fossa is located in the anterior aspect of the elbow. It forms a triangle, the base of which is formed by an imaginary line drawn through the two epicondyles. The lateral border of the fossa is formed by the medial border of the brachioradialis muscle, and the medial border is formed from the lateral border of the pronator teres muscle. Moving from a lateral to medial direction the fossa contains:

- the tendon of biceps (T)
- the brachial artery (A)
- the median nerve (N)

The Carrying Angle

With the arm at the side and the forearm supinated, it can be seen that the forearm forms a valgus angle of between 10-15°. This is the "carrying angle," and it is greater in women than in men.

If the elbow is flexed it can be seen that the valgus position in extension becomes a varus one in flexion. The loss of the valgus position as the elbow moves toward flexion is thought to be due to the varying lip of the trochlea (Tullos & Bryan, 1985).

Note should be taken of the switch from a valgus to varus position as the elbow moves from extension to flexion by watching the position change in the supinated hand (Tullos & Bryan, 1985).

ARTHROKINEMATICS OF THE ELBOW COMPLEX

This is a compound joint consisting of **the humeroradial joint** and **the humeroulnar joint**. In addition, the capsule embraces the **superior radioulnar joint** which, though not part of the true elbow joint, is nevertheless intimately related to it.

The Humeroradial Joint

The close packed position is semiflexion and semipronation. The loose packed position is extension and supination.

The articular surfaces involved in the formation of this joint are the capitulum of the humerus and the facet on the superior aspect of the head of the radius. The joint is involved in flexion and extension of the elbow, but it plays a role in pronation and supination. During flexion and extension, the articular surface of the radius moves in the same direction as the bone, that is, in an anterior direction with flexion and a posterior direction with extension. This direction is in accordance with the concave convex rule, since the articular surface of the superior aspect of the radius is concave.

The Humeroulnar Joint

The close packed position of this joint is extension and the loose packed position is semiflexion.

This joint is formed by the trochlea of the humerus and the trochlear notch of the ulna. It is primarily concerned with flexion and extension of the elbow. The trochlear fossa of the ulna is concave and hence the articular surface will move in the same direction as the bone.

In addition, there is slight medial and lateral sliding of the ulna which facilitates full range of motion in extension and flexion (Kisner & Colby, 1990). This sliding causes a valgus angulation with extension and a varus angulation with flexion.

The Superior Radioulnar Joint

This joint consists of a convex radial head articulating with the concave radial notch on the lateral side of the proximal part of the ulna. Integrally associated with this joint is the annular ligament, which embraces the head of the radius and is attached to the posterior and anterior aspects of the notch. The latter is lined with articular cartilage, and this is continuous with that lining the annular ligament (Norkin & Levangie, 1983).

The Inferior Radioulnar Joint

Although this joint is not part of the elbow complex, it is nevertheless linked to the superior radioulnar joint in terms of function and it is, therefore, appropriate to discuss it here. The concave surface is the ulnar notch on the distal medial aspect of the radius which articulates with the convex head of the ulna. The two bones are joined together by the interosseous membrane.

Pronation and supination are achieved by virtue of the radius crossing and uncrossing over the ulna. At the superior radioulnar joint, the head of the radius spins within the annular ligament and on the radial notch of the ulna. As would be expected from the concave convex rule, the convex radial head slides in a dorsal direction during pronation and a ventral direction during supination. At the inferior radioulnar joint the radius (concave surface) slides over the ulnar head in the same direction in which the bone is moving. It is followed by the articular disc which twists at its apex and sweeps along the ulnar head (Norkin & Levangie, 1983).

DETAILED EXAMINATION

Functional Tests

To test the function of the elbow complex, passive physiological movements are first performed followed by resisted isometric contractions and accessory movements.

Passive Physiological Movements

The physiological movements tested passively are (a) flexion, (b) extension, (c) supination, and (d) pronation. The first two movements occur at the humeroulnar and humeroradial joints, and the last two movements take place at the superior and inferior radioulnar joints.

As indicated earlier, pain or limitation on the performance of a passive movement usually implicates an inert structure.

Isometric Contractions

The isometric contractions tested involve the muscles associated with (a) flexion, (b) extension, (c) supination, and (d) pronation.

With these movements note is made of the following responses: strong and pain free, strong and painful, weak and painful, and weak and pain free. An interpretation of these responses has been provided in Chapters 2 and 3.

Passive Accessory Movements

The passive accessory movements occurring at the elbow complex are (a) traction at the humeroradial joint, (b) dorsal and volar glides of the head of the radius on the humerus, (c) medial and lateral glides of the ulna on the humerus, and (d) dorsal and ventral glides of the head of the radius on the ulna.

Humeroradial Joint

Traction (Figure 6-1)

- *Purpose:* To test for mobility of the radial head.
- *Position of patient:* The patient is in the supine position with the upper arm resting on the plinth; the forearm is supinated and the elbow flexed about 70°.
- *Position of therapist:* The therapist stands with his or her body between the plinth and the patient's forearm and with his or her back to the patient.
- *Proximal grip (fixating grip):* The therapist's right hand is placed on the lower part of the humerus which is fixed firmly in place.
- *Distal grip (mobilizing grip):* The therapist's left hand grips the lower part of the radius, with the thumb on the ventral surface and the fingers on the dorsal surface.
- *Procedure:* The therapist applies traction to the lower part of the radius rotating his or her hips a little to the left as the traction is applied.

Dorsal and Volar Glides of the Head of the Radius on the Humerus (Figure 6-2)

- *Purpose:* To determine the presence of restriction in flexion (volar glide).
- *Position of patient:* The patient is supine, lying with the forearm supinated and the elbow extended. A small pillow, or towel, is placed beneath the lower humerus.
- *Position of therapist:* The therapist stands facing the patient at the level of the elbow.
- *Proximal grip:* The therapist's right hand stabilizes the lower part of the humerus from the medial side.
- *Distal grip:* The heel of the therapist's left hand is placed on the volar aspect of the head of the radius with the fingers embracing the dorsal aspect.
- *Procedure:* The therapist's left hand thrusts down on the radial head to produce a dorsal glide. The fingers lift the radial head anteriorly to produce a ventral glide.

The Humeroulnar Joint

Medial glide of the Ulna

- *Purpose:* This can be used as a test movement to determine whether or not restriction is present. It can also be

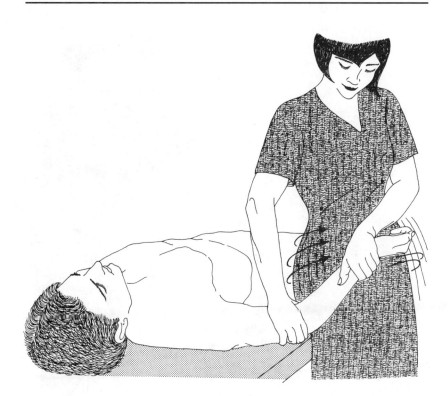

Figure 6-1. Traction of the humeroradial joint.

used as a mobilizing technique to facilitate flexion and extension.

- *Position of the patient:* The patient is in the sitting position with the arm supported near the edge of the plinth. The elbow is in the resting position, with the hand resting gently against the therapist's chest.
- *Position of therapist:* The therapist stands facing the patient.
- *Proximal grip (stabilizing hand):* The therapist's right hand embraces the lower part of the patient's arm, from the medial side, just above the elbow.
- *Distal grip:* The web space between index finger and the thumb of the therapist's left hand is placed against the upper radius, with the remainder of the hand resting on the upper forearm.
- *Procedure:* The medial glide is achieved by the therapist moving the forearm in a medial direction.

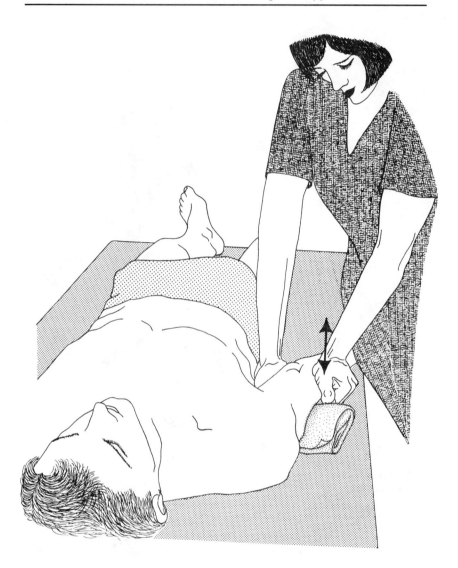

Figure 6-2. Dorsal and volar glides of the head of the radius.

Lateral Glide of Ulna

The position of the patient and the therapist are the same as for the medial glide. The grips are reversed so that the therapist's left hand embraces the lateral aspect of the lower part of the patient's arm. The therapist's right hand is in contact with the upper forearm on the medial side. The glide is achieved by moving the forearm in a lateral direction.

The Superior Radioulnar Joint

Dorsal and Ventral Glides of the Head of the Radius on Ulna

- *Purpose:* To detect restriction of motion in supination (volar glide) and in pronation (dorsal glide).
- *Position of the patient:* The patient is in the sitting position at the side of the plinth with the elbow flexed about 70° and with the forearm (volar surface) resting on the plinth.
- *Position of the therapist:* The therapist stands on the medial side of the patient's forearm with his or her back to the patient's corresponding chest wall.
- *Proximal grip (stabilizing hand):* The therapist's right hand embraces the upper part of the ulna and the lower part of the humerus.
- *Distal grip:* The thumb of the therapist's left hand makes contact with the head of the radius medially, while the flexed index finger makes contact with the head of the radius laterally.
- *Procedure:* The therapist glides the head of the radius in a dorsal-lateral direction by applying pressure with the thumb and in a ventral-medial direction by thrusting with the flexed index finger.

The Inferior Radioulnar Joint Passive accessory movements for this joint are discussed in Chapter 7.

Special Tests

Two special tests will further aid in diagnosis.

Abduction Stress Test

- *Purpose:* To stress the medial collateral ligament of the elbow.
- *Position of the patient:* The patient is in the sitting position with the arm outstretched, the elbow is flexed about 30°, and the forearm is fully supinated.
- *Position of the therapist:* Standing, facing the patient.

- *Proximal grip (stabilizing hand):* The therapist's left hand grips the lower aspect of the humerus and upper aspect of the radius on the lateral side.
- *Distal grip:* The therapist's right hand grips the lower part of the forearm on the medial side.
- *Procedure:* The therapist applies a valgus force (abduction) with the distal hand at the same time that he or she tunes in to the end feel.
- *Interpretation:* Under normal circumstances, a normal capsular end feel should be detected. Note is also taken of the patient's response to the stress test in terms of pain or no pain. If the former is indicated in the presence of a normal end feel, a first-degree sprain of the ligament should be suspected. Increased laxity compared with the other side would indicate a second- or third-degree sprain. (In a first-degree sprain few fibers are torn, many more are torn in a second-degree sprain, and complete disruption of the ligament occurs in a third-degree sprain.)

Adduction Stress Test

- *Purpose:* To stress the lateral collateral ligament.
- *Positions of the patient and therapist:* These are the same as for the medial collateral ligament.
- *Grips:* These are reversed from those described in the previous test.
- *Procedure:* The therapist applies a varus force with the distal hand.
- *Interpretation:* The same as for the medial collateral ligament but applied to the lateral collateral ligament.

SUMMARY

This chapter dealt with the surface anatomy of the elbow complex and the arthrokinematics associated with each joint within the complex. Next, a detailed examination including passive physiological movements, isometric contractions, accessory movements, and special tests was described.

CHAPTER 7

The Wrist and Hand

It has been mentioned in previous chapters that the main function of the upper extremity is to place the hand appropriately in space to facilitate the performance of its many functions. Thus, the shoulder joint is able, via its associated muscular activity, to position the arm in space; similarly the elbow joint is able to move the hand toward the body during flexion and away from the body during extension and the radio-ulnar joints are able to adapt the approach of the hand toward an object (Norkin & Levangie, 1983). Finally, the hand is concerned with precision adjustment (Riordan, 1983) which is necessary for the different functions of the hand (Figure 7-1).

SURFACE ANATOMY

Figure 7-2 shows the carpal bones and bones of the hand that will be discussed in the following paragraphs.

Radius and Ulna

With the patient's hand in the palm down position in space, the radial and ulnar styloids of the patient's right wrist can be palpated. The therapist places his or her left thumb on the

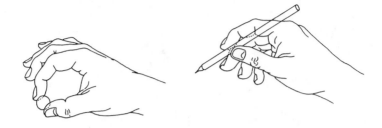

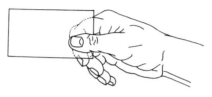

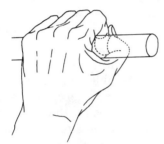

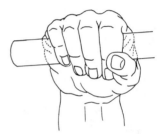

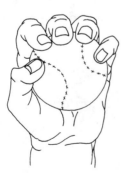

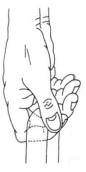

Figure 7-1. Functions of the hand.

side of the lowest part of the radius and the index finger on the side of the lowest part of the ulna, making a squeezing motion. The radial styloid extends two centimeters distal to the styloid of the ulna (Backhouse & Hutchings,1986).

Proximal Row of Carpals

The proximal row of carpals includes, moving from a lateral to a medial direction, the scaphoid, lunate, triquetrum, and pisiform.

The patient's right hand is placed in the palm down position in space with the forearm resting on the plinth. The therapist supports the patient with his or her right hand just above the wrist. The patient is asked to move the thumb laterally away from the index finger (i.e., extend it). An indentation can be seen just distal to the radial styloid. This indentation is called the **"anatomical snuff box."**

The therapist places his or her thumb deeply into this indentation. The **scaphoid**, situated in the proximal row of carpals, and forming the floor of the "anatomical snuff box," can be palpated. The tubercle on the scaphoid can be palpated on the palmar aspect of the hand if the therapist places the index finger on the distal part of the thenar eminence and squeezes the scaphoid between index finger and thumb. The tubercle becomes more prominent if the wrist is deviated in a radial direction (Backhouse & Hutchings, 1986).

With the patient's hand in the palm up position and by moving directly medially from the scaphoid, the therapist can pinch the **lunate** bone between the index finger on the dorsum of the hand and the thumb on the palmar aspect. This is a more mobile structure than the scaphoid.

Still moving in a medial direction, a pea-shaped structure can be palpated just distal to the ulnar styloid. This is the **pisiform** bone lying on top of the triquetrum. Thus palpation of the proximal row of carpals is now completed.

Distal Row of Carpals

The distal row of carpals includes the hamate, capitate, trapezoid, and trapezium. These bones can be readily palpated.

The patient's right hand is in the palm down position in space with the forearm resting on the plinth and the wrist in a few degrees of flexion.The therapist is facing the patient and supports the patient's forearm with his or her left hand placed just above the wrist. The thumb of the therapist's right hand locates the third metacarpal and traces it proximally to its base. Just proximal to the base of the third metacarpal there is an indentation which is the landmark for locating the **capitate** bone. The latter can be palpated between the therapist's thumb on the dorsal aspect and the index finger on the palmar aspect.

If the therapist moves his or her thumb and index finger in an ulnar direction to the base of the fourth and fifth metacarpals, the **hamate** bone can be palpated. The hook of the hamate lies a centimeter distally and radially above the pisiform and is best palpated with the patient's hand in the palm up position and the therapist's thumb pressing deeply into the hypothenar eminence at this level. Note that the pisiform and the hook of hamate lie in a direct diagonal line with the web space between the thumb and index finger (Hoppenfeld, 1976).

With the patient's hand palm down, the therapist places his or her right thumb on the capitate on the dorsum of the patient's distal row of carpals. From this position, the thumb is moved in a radial direction just proximal to the base of the second metacarpal where the **trapezoid** bone can be palpated. This is achieved by utilizing a pinch grip between the thumb on the dorsal aspect of the hand and the index finger on the palmar aspect. Finally, by moving the thumb again in a radial direction proximal to the base of the thumb, the **trapezium** can be palpated.

It is worth noting that if the dorsal surface of the third metacarpal is traced in a proximal direction it will pass over the capitate, lunate, and **Lister's tubercle** (Hoppenfeld, 1976). The latter is a tubercle on the dorsal aspect of the radius just proximal to the proximal row of carpals.

ARTHROKINEMATICS OF THE WRIST JOINT AND THE MIDCARPAL JOINT

The arthrokinematics of the wrist joint and midcarpal joint are complex and controversial, particularly in terms of the role of

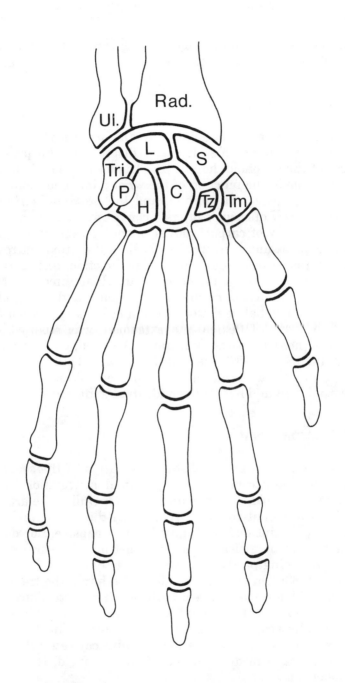

Figure 7-2. The carpal bones and bones of the hand.

the carpus. Some differing opinions regarding the arthrokinematics of these bones are presented below.

The Radiocarpal (Wrist) Joint

This joint is formed proximally by the undersurface of the radius and the radioulnar disc and distally by the proximal surfaces of the scaphoid, lunate, and triquetrum. The ulna does not play a role in the function of the wrist joint. The radius and disc offer a concave articulation, and the proximal surface of the proximal row of carpals offers a convex surface. As a result, the proximal row of carpals moves in the opposite direction to the hand; for example, in wrist extension, the proximal row of carpals can be seen to move in a volar direction, and in radial deviation they are seen to move in an ulnar direction. More flexion than extension occurs at this joint and more ulnar deviation than radial deviation (Norkin & Levangie, 1983). The reverse, in terms of flexion and extension, was reported in a study of 55 normal wrists (Saraffian, Melamed, & Goshgarian, 1977). Kaltenborn (1989) has stated that with both flexion and dorsiflexion of the hand half the movement occurs at the radiocarpal joint and half at the midcarpal joint.

The Midcarpal Joint

This joint is formed by the distal articulation of the scaphoid, lunate, and triquetrum and the proximal articulation of the trapezium, trapezoid, capitate, and hamate. Unlike the articulation of the proximal row of carpals with the radius and disc, the midcarpal joint does not have its own capsule, nor does it form a consistent articular surface. Instead, the surface is a sinuous one, being partly concave and partly convex (Norkin & Levangie, 1983). On the radial side of the hand, the trapezium and trapezoid form a concave surface which articulates with the convex surface formed by the lateral distal articulating surface of the scaphoid. On the ulnar side of the hand, the convex surface formed by the hamate and capitate articulates with the concave medial surface of the scaphoid, the lunate, and triquetrum.

As the proximal row of carpals moves in an ulnar direction in radial deviation, the distal row of carpals moves in the opposite direction (Voltz, Lieb, & Benjamin, 1980). However, it has been reported that the distal row of carpals locks into the proximal row during radial and ulnar deviation, thus ensuring that the two rows move as one and that the midcarpal joint contributes to flexion and extension only (MacConaill & Basmajian, 1977).

DETAILED EXAMINATION

Observation

Swelling can be found in any part of the wrist or hand; it may be the result of trauma, a rheumatological condition, a fracture, or an overuse syndrome. It may be local or general in nature.

Atrophy can develop as a result of a peripheral nerve lesion, a nerve root lesion, or from disuse.

Discoloration may indicate an autonomic problem, ecchymosis, or a skin disorder.

Deformity may occur at the wrist or in the fingers as a result of a fracture, a rheumatological disorder, or a crush or laceration injury.

Resting Position of the hand can be observed by asking the patient to place the dorsum of the hand in a relaxed position on a table. It will be noted that the degree of flexion of the fingers increases from a radial to ulnar direction.

Normal Tenodesis Action can be determined by first asking the patient to extend the wrist; the fingers should flex. Then ask the patient to flex the wrist and the fingers should extend.

Normal Alignment can be verified by observing the alignment of the nails with the fingers in easy flexion; they should be parallel to each other.

Rotational Alignment can be verified by asking the patient to bend the little finger down into the palm; it should point directly to the tuberosity of the scaphoid as will all the fingers if flexed independently. When the fingers are flexed altogether they will lie over the area proximal to the tuberosity of the scaphoid.

Note: Although painful symptoms arising from a local focus in the hand do not usually radiate, it must be remembered that the cervical nerve roots from C5 to T1 can refer pain and parethesia to the wrist and hand. However, careful performance of the upper quadrant scan examination would help to eliminate these structures as the source of the patient's pain.

Functional Tests

These involve passive movements to test the inert joint structures, resisted isometric contractions to test the integrity of the muscles involved in joint movements, accessory movements to test the small articular movements, and special tests used to detect or confirm abnormalities.

Passive Movements

These are described below under the different joint headings.

Inferior Radioulnar Joint The inferior radioulnar joint, although not part of the wrist and hand, is included in the examination process because problems involving the capsule of this joint can cause pain in the wrist. The two movements performed are pronation and supination.

Radiocarpal Joint (True Wrist Joint) The passive movements performed are flexion, extension, and radial and ulnar deviation.

1st Carpometacarpal Joint This joint is formed by the trapezium in the distal row of carpals and the base of the first metacarpal. This joint is commonly affected by arthritis, and to detect the presence of this common malady, the passive movement of extension is performed. This movement stretches the anterior capsule causing pain in the presence of arthritis.

Resisted Isometric Contractions

These are identified below under the different joint headings.

Radiocarpal Joint The contractions achieved against resistance are flexion, extension, and radial and ulnar deviation.

1st Carpometacarpal Joint The contractions achieved against resistance are flexion, extension, abduction, and adduction.

Fingers The contractions achieved individually against resistance are abduction and adduction; those contractions performed collectively are flexion and extension.

Note: To test extrinsic extensors, the MCPs are extended with IP flexion; to test intrinsic extensors, the IPs are extended with MCP flexion.

Accessory Movements

Inferior Radioulnar Joint This joint was mentioned in the previous chapter. It takes part in the movements of pronation and supination in conjunction with the superior radioulnar joint.

Dorsal-Volar Glide (Figure 7-3)

- *Purpose:* To test for restriction of pronation or supination.
- *Position of patient:* Sitting; forearm supported and supinated 10°.
- *Position of therapist:* Standing, facing patient's hand.
- *Fixating grip:* Right hand fixes distal end of ulna between thumb on ventral surface and index on dorsal surface.

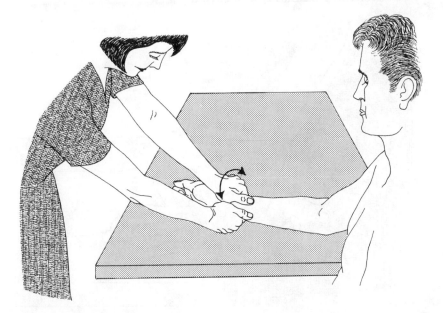

Figure 7-3. Dorsal and volar glides of the radius on the ulna at the distal radioulnar joint.

- *Mobilizing grip:* Left hand holds distal end of radius between thumb ventrally and index dorsally.
- *Procedure:* The radius is moved in a dorsal or ventral direction.

Radiocarpal Joint *Note:* For all accessory movements, the radiocarpal joint should be positioned in some degrees of flexion, which is the "loose-packed" position.

Traction (Figure 7-4)

- *Purpose:* To test general mobility of the wrist joint.
- *Position of patient:* The patient sits with the forearm in space and the elbow flexed; the hand is in the resting or "loose-packed" position.
- *Position of therapist:* The therapist stands by the side of the patient.
- *Proximal grip:* Firmly round the lowest part of the radius and ulna.
- *Distal grip:* The web between the index and first finger of the therapist's right hand fits as closely as possible to the web of the therapist's left hand. The right hand should be over the proximal row of carpals.

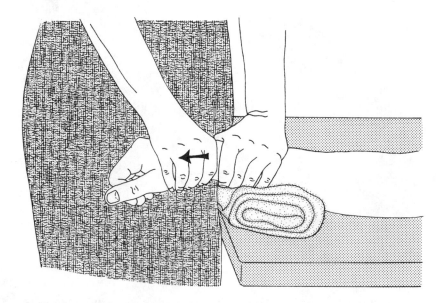

Figure 7-4. Traction to the radiocarpal joint.

- *Procedure:* The therapist applies traction to the proximal row of carpals.

Ventral Glide (Figure 7-5)

- *Purpose:* To detect restriction that would affect the range of extension at the wrist.
- *Position of patient:* The patient sits at the end of the plinth with the forearm pronated and supported, but the wrist clear of the plinth.
- *Position of therapist:* The therapist stands at the side of the patient.
- *Proximal (fixating) grip:* Firmly over the lowest part of the radius and ulna.
- *Distal (mobilizing) grip:* As close to the proximal grip as possible and over the proximal row of carpals.
- *Procedure:* The therapist applies gentle traction and then eases the proximal row of carpals in a volar direction with his or her mobilizing hand.

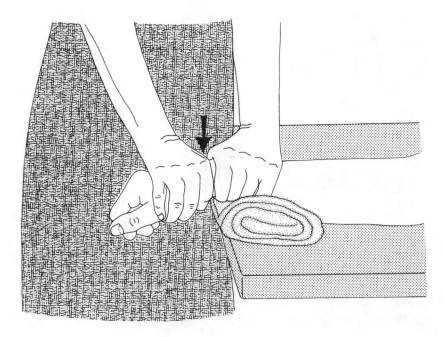

Figure 7-5. Ventral glide of the carpals at the radiocarpal joint.

Dorsal Glide (Figure 7-6)

- *Purpose:* To detect any restriction that may affect flexion of the wrist.
- *Position of patient and therapist:* The position of the therapist and the patient are the same as for the ventral glide except that the patient's forearm is supinated and the palm of the hand is looking upwards.
- *Proximal grip:* This is the same as the proximal grip in the ventral glide.
- *Distal grip:* The therapist's right hand moves in over the volar surface of the proximal row of carpals as close as possible to the proximal grip. At the same time, the therapist holds the patient's wrist in some degrees of flexion.
- *Procedure:* The therapist applies slight traction and glides the proximal row of carpals in a dorsal direction.

Glides to Facilitate Radial and Ulnar Deviation (Figure 7-7)

- *Position of patient:* The patient sits at the end of the plinth with the forearm supported and supinated 10°.

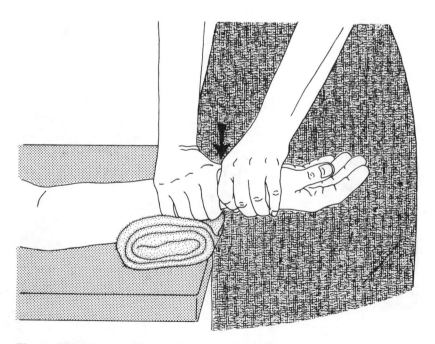

Figure 7-6. Dorsal glide of the carpals at the radiocarpal joint.

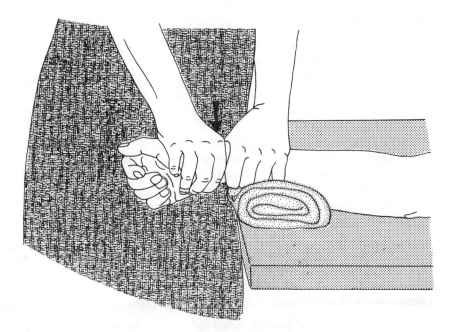

Figure 7-7. Ulnar glide of the carpals at the radiocarpal joint.

- *Grips:* As described for the dorsal glide, except that the index finger of the therapist's right hand is on the volar surface of the proximal row of carpals; the thumb embraces the dorsal surface.
- *Procedure:* The therapist applies slight traction as he or she glides the proximal row of carpals in an ulnar direction to facilitate radial deviation. To facilitate ulnar deviation, the forearm is pronated so that the radial side of the forearm lies in contact with the plinth, and the wrist is clear of it. With the wrist in this position, the therapist glides the proximal row of carpals in a radial direction.

Special Tests

Abnormal vascular, synovial, connective, or muscular tissues may be the cause of pain and/or stiffness, and can be specifically tested. The following tests are commonly used in the assessment of the hand.

The Allen Test

- *Purpose:* To determine the efficacy of the blood flow in the radial and ulnar arteries.
- *Procedure:* The patient is instructed to make a fist then release it several times. Next he or she is requested to make a fist and hold it so that the venous blood is forced from the palm.

  The therapist locates the radial artery with his or her thumb and the ulnar artery with the index and middle fingers. Pressure is exerted on these arteries to occlude them and the patient is asked to open his or her hand. The therapist releases the pressure on one of the arteries and watches for immediate flushing. If this does not occur, or the response is slow, there is interference in the normal blood supply to the hand. The procedure is repeated for the other artery.

Finkelstein's Test

- *Purpose:* This test is used to determine whether pain experienced in the region of the radial styloid is due to inflammation of the synovial sheath surrounding extensor pollicis brevis and abductor pollicis longus (De Quervain's disease).
- *Procedure:* The patient's thumb is flexed across the palm, and the hand is deviated in an ulnar direction. A painful response is indicative of involvement of the sheath.

The Bunnel-Littler Test

- *Purpose:* This test is used to determine whether the presence of restricted flexion of the proximal interphalangeal joint is due to tightness of the intrinsics or tightness of the joint capsule.
- *Procedure:* The metacarpophalangeal joint is placed in a few degrees of extension, just beyond the neutral position and the therapist attempts to flex the proximal interphalangeal joint. Restriction of flexion in this joint can either be due to tightness of the intrinsics or of the joint capsule.

  The metacarpophalangeal joint is then placed in a few degrees of flexion to release the intrinsics, and an attempt is made to flex the proximal interphalangeal joint. If full flexion cannot be achieved at this joint, tightness of the joint capsule must be suspected.

The Retinacular Test

- *Purpose:* To determine whether restriction of flexion in the distal interphalangeal joint is due to a tight retinaculum or a tight capsule.
- *Procedure:* The proximal interphalangeal joint is flexed a few degrees to relax the retinaculum. If the restriction of flexion still remains, the restriction in flexion at the distal phalangeal joint is due to a tight capsule.

SUMMARY

In this chapter, pertinent bony landmarks were identified and the controversial aspects of the arthrokinematics of the midcarpal joint were discussed. The detailed examination began with observation of significant aspects relating to the hand and its alignment. During the detailed examination the physiological movements, isometric contractions, accessory movements, as well as special tests were applied to the major joints and muscles of the wrist and hand.

CHAPTER 8

• • • • • • • •

Lower Quadrant Screening Examination (SCAN)

The lower quadrant screening examination is similar to that of the upper quadrant screening examination. Following the subjective examination the areas examined are the lumbar spine, the peripheral joints of the lower limb, the myotomes of the lumbar nerve roots and those of S1 and S2, the dermatomes, and the reflexes of the lower limb.

SUBJECTIVE EXAMINATION

Patient's Medical History

The principles outlined in the subjective examination in Chapter 3 are pursued here and the reader is advised to review that chapter. Questions regarding the location, type, extent, severity, and behavior of the patient's pain must be asked. Of particular interest in the lower quadrant scan are symptoms such as:

- paresthesia and its location (the saddle area has grave significance).
- any problems with micturition.
- weakness of the legs, or an unsteady gait.

111

In the scenario in Chapter 3, it was assumed that the patient was suffering from shoulder pain. In the following scenario the patient is suffering from pain in the low back, but it could be anywhere in the lower extremity or perhaps in both areas. Let us follow through with a typical scenario for a patient with a problem in the lower quadrant.

Scenario

Once again for the sake of clarity and comprehension it is assumed that the patient is ideal and that her responses are clear and to the point. The guidelines for asking questions on page 31 should be reviewed, since they apply here also.

Q.1. "Can you show me where you feel the pain?"
(The patient places her hand on the low back).

Q.2. "Is the pain there all the time?"

A. "No."

Q.3. "Do you have pain now?"

A. "No."

Q.4. "When did you last have the pain?"

A. "Last night. I'd been putting the plants in the garden and was rather tired, so I thought I'd sit and watch TV. I watched a movie, but my back began to bother me."

Q.5. "Did you feel the pain when you were in the garden?"

A. "No, it came on later when I was watching TV."

Q.6. "Can you describe the pain for me?"

A. "It's an ache."

Q.7. "How would you rate the ache on a scale of one to ten?"

A. "Five most of the time, but if I don't move around it can be much worse."

Q.8. "You said you felt the ache when you were sitting watching TV. What happened then?"

A. "I went to bed."

Q.9. "What happened to your ache when you were in bed?"

A. "It went away; it always does if I lie down."

Q.10. "When did you have the pain before last night?"

A. "It niggles on and off during the day, but the last time it really ached was a couple of days ago when

I drove down from the cottage. Again I had been busy mowing the grass and raking up leaves before I left."

Q.11. "Are you aware of anything you do which brings on the ache?"

A. "Well, it seems to come on if I've been busy working at something, like the garden, and then sit down to relax."

Q.12. "Does it come on at any time other than when you are sitting?"

A. "Now that I think about it I always seem to get the ache after sitting for any length of time."

Note in the scenario how the patient wants to associate her back pain with some activity, but the therapist's questions elicit the fact that the ache only comes on when she sits down to relax following an activity.

The therapist would continue the questioning regarding the length of time the patient has had the problem, whether she has had back ache before and whether she has other musculoskeletal problems. The general state of the patient's health would be determined and the type of medication the patient is presently taking would also be determined. In addition, her age, occupation, and recreational activities would be ascertained.

Mandatory Questions

These have been mentioned before, but are worthy of reiteration here. The therapist must determine whether the patient is on:

- a prolonged course of corticosteroid medication (this can cause osteoporosis).
- anticoagulants (may make the patient vulnerable to hemarthrosis).
- analgesics and anti-inflammatory drugs (can influence signs and symptoms).

It is also important for the therapist to know if the patient has had ankylosing spondylitis or any other inflammatory condition that may weaken the ligaments of the lumbar spine. If the patient has had cancer, the therapist must be alerted to the possibility of metastases; or if the patient had radiation in the region, this could cause osteoporosis (Magarey, 1988).

OBJECTIVE EXAMINATION

Observation

When observing a patient with a problem in the lower quadrant, the therapist is again concerned with deviations from the normal posture. The first observation takes place as the patient walks. Is there an antalgic gait? What is the patient's dynamic posture? Then note is taken of the patient's static posture. Is the patient standing erect and exhibiting the normal curvatures of the spinal column? The general observation also takes in the lower limbs, and each limb is compared with the other for muscle bulk and positional deviations. The levels of the bony landmarks are of particular importance. A number of asymmetries have no clinical significance; however, it is important to record any deviation from the norm.

Standing Position

The patient stands with the feet placed hip width apart.

Anterior Aspect The patient is in the standing position facing the therapist.

Anterior Superior Iliac Spines (ASIS): These can be compared by the examiner getting down to eye level and placing a thumb on each ASIS.
Iliac Crests: These are compared as the therapist's hands approach from the lateral aspect of the ilia in a cephalic direction and move inwards so that the ventral aspect of the fingers come to rest on the iliac crests.
Patellae: The level and position of the patellae are noted and compared. Are they looking straight ahead?
Knees: Is there evidence of genu valgum or varum?
Feet: Are the feet pointing straight ahead? Is there any evidence of a pronated or supinated foot?

Lateral Aspect. Here the examiner is taking note of:

Head: Is there a forward head posture?
Trunk: Is there a forward lean? Is there any evidence of

a thoracic kyphosis or an excessive lumbar lordosis?
Hips and Knees: Are there any signs of flexion contractures, recurvatum, and so on?

Posterior Aspect Many patients with low back pain will lean
away from the affected side, producing a lumbar scoliosis or
lateral shift (McKenzie, 1981). The therapist will observe for
lateral deviations of the spinal column as well as soft tissue
deviations. The patient may present with a lumbar or thoracic
kyphosis and this should be noted.

Posterior Superior Iliac Spines (PSIS): The therapist
places his or her thumbs just below the dimples located
near the posterior extreme of the iliac crests and
compares the level of one side with the other.
Knee Creases: The creases on the posterior aspect of the
patient's knees are compared.
Tendoachilles: Do the tendons fall in a straight line or
are they going into varus or valgus?

The observation of the posterior aspect is completed by
taking note of swelling, abrasions, atrophy, or any other
abnormality.

Functional Testing

Spinal Movements

These movements are forward flexion, extension in standing,
side flexion in standing, and rotation in sitting.

Forward Flexion This is performed in the standing position.
The patient is asked to run the fingers down the front of the
legs as far as possible with comfort. Range and comfort of
performance are noted. If the movement is full and pain free,
overpressure (OP) is applied.

Notice is taken of the presence of any deviation to the right
or left during the performance of this movement. This is
suggestive of a restricting problem in the lumbar spine
(McKenzie, 1981). The therapist also takes note of the reversal
of the lumbar spine as it goes from the lordotic position in
standing to the flexed position. If reversal of the curve does not
occur and the spine remains flat, bilateral muscle spasm may
be the causative factor. The patient may veer toward one side

as forward flexion is performed and then correct as forward flexion continues. Finally, note is taken of the thoracic spine as it goes into flexion. If it does not straighten out properly, a rib hump may be present, which is indicative of a structural scoliosis.

Extension in Standing The patient places the hands in the small of the back and extends the spine. Once again, range and comfort of performance is noted; if pain free, OP is applied.

Side Flexion in Standing The patient is encouraged to bend to one side maintaining the trunk in the neutral position. Note is taken of the level of the patient's fingers on the lateral aspect of the patient's thigh or leg. Comparison is made between the right and left side. Once again, on completion of a pain free movement, OP is applied.

Rotation in Sitting The patient sits on a stool with the hands on opposite shoulders and performs rotation as far to the right as possible. If the movement does not cause pain OP is applied. The movement is then repeated to the left.

Peripheral Joints

In the following passive movement tests, the therapist takes note of the end feel at the end of range.

1. *Hip.* The therapist passively moves the patient's right hip into abduction stabilizing the left hip as he or she does so.
2. *Knee.* Passive flexion and extension are performed.
3. *Ankle.* Passive dorsi and plantar flexion are performed.
4. *Midtarsal Joint.* Movement at the ankle joint is restricted while the therapist inverts and everts the foot at the midtarsal joint.
5. *Subtalar Joint.* The therapist cups the patient's heel in his or her hands, applies a little traction to fix the talus, and inverts and everts the heel.

Myotomes

The following testing procedure is similar to that performed in the upper quadrant in that attempts are made to produce a strong isometric contraction in each myotome. The therapist requests the patient to hold the limb in a given position and not let the therapist move it.

1. *L2. Iliopsoas* The patient is in the lying position with the hip and knee flexed to 90°. The therapist sits sideways on the plinth with the calf of the patient's leg resting on her shoulder. The therapist's hands are interlocked around the patient's anterior thigh and as he or she attempts to extend the patient's thigh the patient resists the movement.
2. *L3. Quadriceps* The therapist tries to bend the patient's knee over his or her arm at the same time as the patient attempts to resist any movement.
3. *L4. Tibialis Anterior* The patient holds the foot in dorsiflexion and inversion as the therapist attempts to plantarflex and evert it.
4. *L5. Extensor Hallucis* The therapist attempts to flex the great toe as the patient resists the movement.
5. *S1. Peronei* The patient holds the foot in eversion as the therapist attempts to invert it.

Sensory and Reflex Testing

The dermatomes (Figures 8-1, 8-2, 8-3) are tested by the therapist by lightly running the pads of the fingers across them in a circuitous fashion. At the same time, the patient is asked to let the therapist know of any change in sensation, such as numbness or hyperesthesia, and so on.

Suspect areas of skin can be further tested utilizing pin pricks or even two-point discrimination. The reflexes of the lower extremity are L3 (ligamentum patellae) and S1 (the tendoachilles). A sluggish response, or no response at all, could be interpreted as interference with nerve root conductivity.

SUMMARY

In this chapter, quick tests for the physiological movements of the lumbar and thoracic spines, the peripheral joints, the myotomes and dermatomes associated with the lumbosacral plexus, and the relevant reflexes have been described.

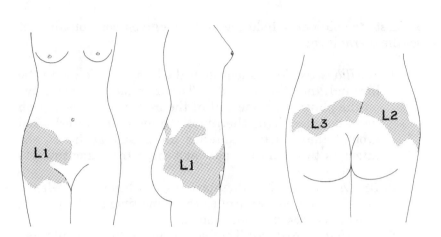

Figure 8-1. Dermatomes for nerve roots L1, L2, and L3.

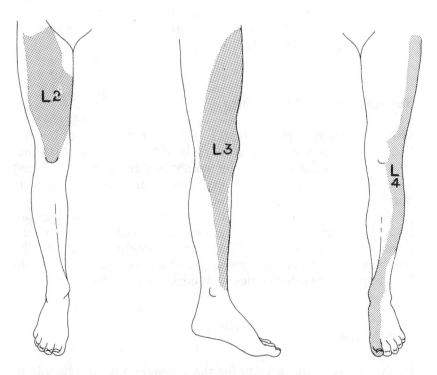

Figure 8-2. Dermatomes for nerve roots L2, L3, and L4.

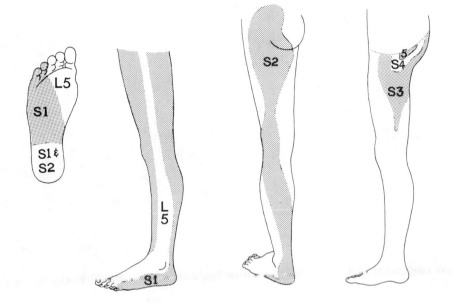

Figure 8-3. Dermatomes for nerve roots L5, S1, S2, S3, S4, and S5.

CHAPTER 9

Detailed Examination of the Thoracolumbar Spine and the McKenzie Examination

The thoracic spine is less vulnerable to injury than the cervical or lumbar spines. Ninety three percent of the disorders of the vertebral column are due to disc degeneration but less than two per cent occur in the thoracic spine (Kramer, 1981). Cloward (1959) and Cyriax (1982) demonstrated that much of the pain experienced in the thoracic region to the level of T7 originated in the cervical spine. For these reasons more time will be devoted, in this chapter, to examination of the lumbar region than the thoracic region.

The thoracic spine is less mobile than the cervical spine because the rib cage is an intimate part of it. However, the bony landmarks are more readily palpable.

BONY LANDMARKS

The Scapula and its Relationship to the Thoracic Vertebrae

The superior angle of the scapula is on the same level as T2 vertebra; the spine of the scapula is on the same level as T3 vertebra, and the inferior angle is on the same level as the spinous process of T7.

Mitchell, Moran, & Pruzzo (1979) divide the thoracic vertebrae into groups of three for the purpose of examination. The spinous processes of the first three thoracic vertebrae (T1, T2, T3) project directly backward; consequently, the tip of the spinous process is on the same line as the transverse processes.

Vertebrae T4, T5, and T6 have spinous processes that project slightly downward; as a result, the tips of these processes are located midway between their own transverse processes and the ones associated with the vertebra below.

The spinous processes of T7, T8, and T9 project moderately downward and are located in line with the transverse processes directly below.

The last three thoracic vertebrae are somewhat more independent than the three sets just described, because as a trio they do not conform. The spinous process of T10 is almost on the same line as the vertebrae below; T11 spinous process is midway between its own transverse processes and those of the vertebra below it. The spinous process of T12 is in line with its own transverse processes.

The Lumbar Spine

The patient should be positioned in the prone position with one or two pillows beneath the abdomen. The arms lie in a relaxed position at the side of the patient and the patient's head is in a neutral position.

L1 to L5 Spinous Processes

These can be identified by approaching them from the sacrum. The therapist places the fingertips of his or her right hand on the lower part of the sacrum and moves upward. The small ridges representing the spinous processes of the sacral vertebrae can be palpated. The therapist's hand continues moving in an upward direction; the first large, bony projection to be palpated is the spinous process of L5. Although the spinous process of L5 can be readily identified from the sacral processes, it is smaller than the other lumbar processes and lies deeper. The remaining spinous processes of the lumbar vertebrae are identified by moving upward. It should be noted that these are quite prominent, each one forming a thick, bony, vertical ridge.

The Facet Joints

The facet joints lie deeply in an area about one inch lateral to the lower tip of the spinous process. They are covered with the paravertebral musculature and are not as easy to palpate as those in the cervical spine.

The Transverse Processes

These are located about half an inch lateral to the facet joints (or about one and a half inches from the spinous processes) and a little inferior. They lie on a line midway between two spinous processes.

The Iliac Crests

The highest part of the crests lies on a level with the interspace between L4 and L5 spinous processes.

The Posterior Superior Iliac Spines (PSIS)

If the iliac crests are followed in a medial and downward direction, two dimples can be identified; below these are the PSIS.

The Sacroiliac Joints (SIJ)

These are formed by the posterior part of the iliac bones and the upper part of the posterolateral aspects of the sacrum.

DETAILED EXAMINATION

Active Movements

These movements have already been covered in the early part of the lower quadrant scan.

Resisted Isometric Contractions

1. **Side flexion:** The therapist stands at the side of the patient applying counter pressure with her or his hip (against the patient's left hip) as the patient attempts to side bend (to the right) against the resistance of the therapist, whose hand is placed on the patient's right upper arm. No isotonic movement occurs. The procedure is repeated when the patient attempts to side bend against resistance to the left.
2. **Rotation:** The therapist's position and that of the patient are the same as for passive rotation. The therapist attempts to rotate the patient first in one direction then the other, instructing the patient: "Don't let me move you, hold." Once again an isometric contraction is achieved.
3. **Forward Flexion:** The patient is sitting over the edge of the plinth (or chair). The therapist is standing on the patient's right side. The therapist applies resistance with the proximal hand over the sternum. The distal hand is placed just above the knees to stabilize the patient. The patient attempts to lean forward against the therapist's resistance, but is not permitted to move.
4. **Extension:** The patient is in the prone position on the plinth. The therapist stands at the side of the patient, the proximal hand is placed on the patient's upper thoracic spine, while the distal hand is placed over the patient's pelvis. The patient attempts to extend the thoracic spine against the therapist's resistance, producing an isometric contraction.

Interpretation of Isometric Contraction Testing

1. **Side Flexion:** Pain here implicates the obliques on the side to which the patient is trying to side flex.
2. **Rotation:** This involves the internal oblique on the side toward which the patient is trying to turn and the external oblique of the opposite side.
3. **Flexion:** This implicates rectus abdominis.
4. **Extension:** The erector spinae would be involved if there is a painful response to this movement.

On completion of the lower quadrant scan examination and the examination of the thoracolumbar spine, most of the examination relating to the spine has been performed. However, the accessory movements involving the thoracic and lumbar spines and special tests (particularly relating to the lumbar spine) need to be performed.

Accessory Movements of the Thoracic and Lumbar Spines

The movements that need to be performed are posteroanterior (PA) pressures on the spinous processes and the transverse processes and transverse pressures against the spinous processes (Maitland, 1986). The performance of these movements help to localize and further identify the patient's problems.

Posteroanterior Pressures on the Spinous Processes and Transverse Processes

Spinous Processes

It is helpful to perform general passive movements with the heel of the hand over several segments at once. These can be performed by the therapist placing the heel of the hand over several spinous processes in the thoracic spine and applying a PA pressure as she or he descends the spine into the lumbar region. Symptoms arising are noted.

Next, to be more specific, the hypothenar eminence of the therapist's right hand is used (with the left hand reinforcing the right) over each spinous process, both in the thoracic and lumbar spines. The response from each segment is noted.

Transverse Processes

The preceding procedure is repeated, but the hypothenar eminence is now placed over the transverse process to produce a rotary movement to the opposite side.

Transverse Pressures Against the
Spinous Processes

The therapist stands at the patient's left side. The therapist's arms are extended so that the elbows are straight, and the pad(s) of the thumbs rest against the side of the spinous process. The therapist performs a transverse movement which produces a rotation towards the side on which the therapist is working.

Special Tests

1. *The Straight Leg Raising Test (SLR Test)* (Urban, 1986). The purpose of this test is to detect an increase in nerve root tension.

- *Position of patient:* The patient is in the supine position with the neck in neutral or slightly extended. The hips should be in neutral, neither abducted or adducted or rotated.
- *Position of therapist:* Standing at the side of the patient.
- *Procedure:* The therapist raises the patient's leg maintaining the limb in the neutral position with the knee extended. The therapist takes note of the site and range of motion at which pain is felt.

   Confirmation that the nerve root is the cause of the patient's pain can be obtained by lowering the limb to the point at which there is no pain and then dorsiflexing the ankle. If pain is reproduced, the nerve root is confirmed as the culprit.

2. *Babinski's Test.* The patient is in the supine position. The therapist draws a sharp object up the sole of the patient's foot. A positive result is present if the great toe extends and the remaining toes spread out. A positive result is indicative of an upper motor neuron lesion.

   Note: Cyriax (1982) has pointed out that it is important to clear the cervical spine in the presence of pain in the upper thoracic region as cervical disc problems are a common cause of posterior upper thoracic pain.

SOME ASPECTS OF THE MCKENZIE EXAMINATION OF THE LUMBAR SPINE

It will be recalled from the McKenzie examination of the cervical spine that specific postures and movements are used to determine what brings on the patient's pain, which movements increase (peripheralize) the pain, and which movements decrease (centralize) the patient's pain. Similarly in assessing the lumbar spine McKenzie (1981) is interested in the patient's posture in sitting and standing and in the utilization of test movements to determine the quality of the movement, and repeated test movements to cause peripheralization of the patient's pain or centralization of the pain.

Observation of the Patient's Posture

A good time to observe the patient's sitting posture is during the subjective examination. The patient will automatically choose the posture that he or she habitually assumes and the therapist has plenty of time to take note of it. The therapist also observes the patient in the standing position for an accentuated or reduced lordosis and for the presence of a lateral shift. This is present if the shoulders and trunk have moved laterally in relation to the pelvis. It is described in terms of the direction of the shift of the shoulders and the trunk; if they have moved to the left this is described as a left lateral shift. When it is present and symptomatic it is indicative of a derangement. Usually the shift develops away from the painful side. It is important to detect even the slightest lateral shift and to correct it if it is contributing to the patient's pain.

Correction of the Lateral Shift

This correction is achieved by the therapist standing on the side of the lateral shift (as described above it would be the left side). The patient is asked to bend his or her left elbow to 90° and to hug the elbow to the side. The therapist bends down and hugs the patient's pelvis so that the therapist's arms are embracing the front and back of the pelvis and the hands are interlocked over the right pelvis. The correction is achieved by the therapist gently easing his or her left shoulder against the patient's left shoulder and thorax a little at a time as he or she eases the patient's right pelvis to the left with the hands. The procedure is repeated until correction of the left lateral shift is achieved. It is important to monitor the patient's pain to avoid exacerbation, and to take time with the corrective process.

Examination of Movement

It is during this part of the examination that the repetitive movements are used; however, the first three movements performed in standing are performed only once to assess the quality of movement. The patient is encouraged to move as far as possible with each movement.

Single Test Movements

1. Flexion: Provides the examiner with the most relevant information regarding the nature and extent of the disturbance in derangement and dysfunction. Ask the patient to bend forward as far as possible by running the fingertips down the front of the legs and returning immediately to the neutral standing position. Loss of flexion manifests itself in two ways
   a. end of range is limited
      • watch for presence of lordosis or flat lumbar spine
   b. deviation from normal pathway of flexion
      • derangement within the joint (the deviation is away from the painful side)
      • dysfunction in joint following repair of damaged structures after derangement
      • dysfunction external to the joint
      • tethered nerve root

2. Extension: Some loss of extension is normal after the age of 40, but its presence should be recorded

• major disc bulging will normally cause the patient to lean away from painful side

3. Side gliding: This is a combination of rotation and side flexion; the patient is asked to move his or her shoulders and pelvis simultaneously in opposite directions

Repetitive Test Movements

The purpose of the repetitive test movements is to identify the movements that decrease the patient's pain and those that increase the patient's pain. The patient is asked to move as far as possible with each movement.

The following movements are performed 5 to 10 times.

1. Forward flexion in standing
2. Repeated forward flexion in standing
3. Extension in standing — the patient places the hands in the small of the back and extends the spine over them
4. Repeated extension in standing
5. Side gliding in standing — the patient moves the pelvis in a horizontal line in one direction and the shoulders in a horizontal line in the opposite direction, first to one side then the other
6. Repeated side gliding in standing
7. Flexion in supine lying — the patient's knees are brought onto the chest, and pressure is applied by the patient passively pulling the knees further into the chest, then releasing the pressures — pressure on, pressure off
8. Repeated flexion in supine lying — pressure on, pressure off
9. Extension in prone lying — the patient passively extends the spine by thrusting back from the extended arm prone lying support position maintaining contact between the pelvis and the plinth as he or she does so
10. Repeated extension in lying — "up and down." Throughout the performance of each exercise, the patient is encouraged to move as far as possible in the given direction and then encouraged to return immediately to the starting position. Following each exercise,

the patient should be asked to describe the effect of the exercise on the pain. If a few (e.g., three or four) repetitions of a particular repeated exercise increase the patient's pain, either by perpheralization or intensity, discontinue the exercise. If there is no change, each of the exercises may be repeated up to ten times.

Relationship of Pain to Movement

During test movements in standing, a normal stress is applied to normal or abnormal tissue. During test movements in lying, a passive stress is added by the patient either by pushing the trunk passively into extension using the arms (as in extension in lying) or by pulling the bent knees further onto the chest with the hands, as in flexion in lying; thus, an abnormal stress is applied to normal or abnormal tissue.

In the former case, no pain should develop because the movement is momentary. In the latter case, mechanical deformation is enhanced and pain is produced. Pain will be decreased or abolished if the movement reduces the mechanical deformation.

If the pain is to be related to movements, repetitive movements must produce a change in the patient's symptoms. Movement will increase or decrease the pain, change its location, or one pain could be abolished and another produced. If no pain is present prior to the performance of the repetitive movements, they may produce the pain complained of. If the movements do not change the patient's symptoms:

- they have not been performed vigorously enough and should be repeated, or
- pain is not of mechanical origin, or
- the lumbar spine is not causing the problems, and some other cause should be sought.

Repetitive Movements

In derangement, the performance of repetitive movements in the direction that increases accumulation of nuclear material will increase pain and cause peripheralization. The performance of movements in the opposite direction will result in centralization or reduction of pain.

Repeated movements which cause pain in the direction that stretches are diagnostic of dysfunction, since shortened structures produce pain at end of range. However, these repeated movements should not make the patient worse; otherwise, tearing of the shortened structures has occurred.

Patients with a postural problem will not have pain with any of the test movements.

Note: When repeated movements applied to painful structures produce less and less pain these structures should be exercised. If more pain is produced, more healing time should be allowed.

Flexion and Extension in Standing vs. Lying

Flexion in lying produces no gravitational stress and the movement begins in the lower lumbar spine and ascends to the upper lumbar spine. In flexion in standing the reverse is the case; movement begins at the upper lumbar spine and descends to the lower lumbar spine. A better flexion stretch is obtained in L5 to S1 in passive flexion in lying. Stretching of L4 to L5 to S1, only occurs when flexion in standing is almost full.

The sciatic nerve is fully stretched in flexion in standing. Enhancement of sciatic pain in standing may be caused by a bulging disc or an adherent root. Enhancement of sciatic pain in lying can only be caused by a bulging disc. (In flexion in lying, the tension is taken off the sciatic nerve and, therefore, pain cannot be caused by an adherent nerve root.) In extension in prone lying, if the pelvis is maintained in contact with the plinth, an increase in extension range is achieved. In extension in standing, the compression forces appear to be sufficient to prevent full end range movement. This indicates that some derangements are too large to be reduced in the presence of compressive forces. Reduction of these derangements becomes possible when the compressive forces are reduced by extension in lying.

SUMMARY

This chapter commenced with the surface anatomy of the thoracolumbar spine followed by active movements and resisted isometric contractions and interpretations of findings. Next, posteroanterior pressures over the spinous processes and transverse processes were described, followed by transverse pressures to the spinous processes. This section was completed by the description of special tests. Finally, the reader was introduced to McKenzie's examination of the lumbar spine including the test movements and their interpretation.

CHAPTER 10

The Sacroiliac Joint and Hip

THE SACROILIAC JOINT

The sacroiliac joint is probably the most controversial in the human body. There is a constant debate regarding the amount of movement, the location of the axes, and the vulnerability of the joint to dysfunction. Certainly, the joint is supported by some very strong ligaments that protect it against excessive forces. Cyriax (1982) believes that lesions of the sacroiliac joint are rare. Maitland (1986) states that the sacroiliac joint "is not a common mechanical source of pain." However, the fact remains that this joint is the object of extensive examinations and tests, some of which will be described later.

Bony Landmarks

Iliac Crests

The patient is in the standing position with his or her back to the therapist. The therapist is in the crouch position so that his or her eyes are level with the area to be observed. The therapist places his or her hands on the patient's hips and moves them in a superior direction to the waist line. The hands are then placed in the palm down position so that the lateral borders of the index fingers are in contact with the waist. From this position, the therapist pushes gently inward and downward so that the adipose tissue is moved from the area, enabling the therapist to make contact with the iliac crests. Are they level? If they are not level place an object (e.g., a piece of wood) of appropriate depth under the foot of the short side to equalize the levels.

Posterior Superior Iliac Spines (PSIS)

These bony prominences are located with the patient and therapist in the same position as taken for iliac crests. By following the iliac crests around to their posterior termination, a dimple can be seen bilaterally. The posterior iliac spines can be palpated by placing the thumbs about one centimeter below the dimple. Are the posterior iliac spines level? Are they in the same plane?

Interpretation: If, after making sure that the iliac crests are level in the manner just described, the therapist finds one iliac crest higher than the other, this is indicative of a dysfunction. If one PSIS is anterior to the other, it means either that the external rotators on the same side are tight, or the internal rotators of the opposite side are tight (Mitchell, Moran, & Pruzzo, 1979).

Care must be taken to ensure that the posterior iliac prominences (PIP) are not mistaken for the PSIS. The former are located on a level with the dimples.

Anterior Superior Iliac Spines (ASIS)

For palpation of these bony prominences, the therapist is in front of the patient in a crouch position for easy observance. The therapist locates the iliac crests in the same way as described previously and locates the ASIS with his or her thumbs at the anterior extreme of the iliac crests. Are they level? Are they in the same plane?

Interpretation: This is a confirmatory test for the PSIS one discussed earlier. If the right PSIS is anteriorly displaced in relation to the left PSIS, it follows that the right ASIS would be similarly displaced and the interpretation would be as for the anteriorly displaced PSIS.

Ischial Tuberosities

These bony structures can be palpated with the patient in the standing position with the feet acetabular distance apart. The therapist places the heels of his or her hands on the inferior gluteal folds then moves the hands superiorly until the tuberosities are located.

Alternatively, each ischial tuberosity can be palpated individually. The patient is in right side lying position with the left hip and knee bent to locate the left ischial tuberosity: then the patient moves to the left side lying position with the right hip and knee bent to locate the right ischial tuberosity.

Now that the major bony landmarks have been identified, some of the tests used to locate the cause of the patient's problem will be discussed.

DETAILED EXAMINATION

Special Tests

The first two tests stress the anterior and posterior ligaments respectively of the SI joint. The remaining tests are used to detect clinical asymmetries of the SI joint.

Anterior Ligament Distraction Test

- *Position of the patient and therapist:* The patient is in the supine position with the therapist standing facing him or her and to the side.
- *Procedure:* The therapist ensures that the patient's pelvis is level, then the therapist places one hand on each ASIS and presses downward and laterally.
- *Interpretation:* If there is a problem with either of the anterior ligaments, there will be a painful response on the corresponding side (Cyriax, 1983).

Alternatively, the patient can be placed in the prone position and pressure applied to the center of the sacrum.

Posterior Ligament Compression Test

- *Position of the patient and the therapist:* The patient is in the side lying position with the therapist behind him or her.
- *Procedure:* The therapist places both hands on the anterior part of the iliac crest and thrusts them toward the floor.
- *Interpretation:* Pain in the region of the SI joint of the uppermost leg indicates a problem with the posterior ligaments on that side. The test is repeated for the opposite side (Cyriax, 1983).

Standing Flexion Test

This test (Lee, 1989; Mitchell, Moran, & Pruzzo, 1979) demonstrates the movement of the ilia on the sacrum.

- *Position of patient and therapist:* The patient is in the standing position with the feet firmly planted under the hips. The therapist is standing behind the patient in the crouched position so that his or her eyes are level with the patient's PSISs.
- *Procedure:* The therapist places his or her thumbs on the lower part of the respective PSIS. The patient is requested to bend down slowly as far as he or she can, during which time the therapist maintains thumb contact with the patient's PSIS on both sides.
- *Interpretation:* The movement should be equal in a superior direction. If one thumb is riding higher than the other there is an abnormality due to the fact that the ilium on that side is locked onto the sacrum and follows it. The restriction is on the side of the increased motion (Mitchell, Moran, & Pruzzo, 1979).

Note: Tight hamstrings on one side can cause a difference in excursion and give a false-positive result (Bourdillon, 1982; Mitchell, Moran & Pruzzo, 1979).

Seated Flexion Test

To stabilize the pelvis and eliminate the possible effect of the tight hamstrings, the flexion test is repeated with the patient in the sitting position (Bourdillon, 1982; Mitchell, Moran, & Pruzzo, 1979).

Right Sacroiliac Fixation Test

- *Position of patient and therapist:* The patient is in the standing position with the weight evenly distributed between both lower extremities. The therapist is in the crouch position behind the patient.
- *Procedure:* The therapist places his or her right thumb over the right PSIS and the left thumb on the median sacral crest (the sacralspinous processes) in line with the level of the right thumb. The patient is asked to bend his or her right hip and knee up toward the chest. (Figure 10-1).
- *Interpretation:* Under normal circumstances, the right thumb moves downward as the patient bends the right hip and knee. If the right thumb moves in an upward direction, the right SI joint is fixed (Kirkaldy-Willis, 1983).

Note: Since most of the hip muscles have their origin on the pelvis, tightness in these muscles on the same side, or weakness on the opposite side, can also produce inequality in the levels of the PSIS (Mitchell, Moran, & Pruzzo, 1979). Steindler (1955) has pointed out that tight adductors on one side can cause an elevation of the ASIS on the affected side, and tight abductors can cause a lowering of the ASIS on the affected side. It is, therefore, essential that the hip muscles be tested for both

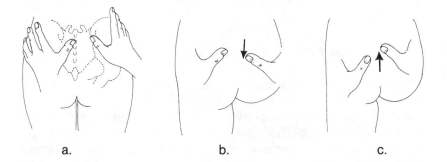

a.   b.   c.

Figure 10-1. The standing hip flexion test for the right SI joint. (a) Position of the examiner's hands; (b) normal response; and (c) indication of a fixed right SI joint. (Adapted from Kirkaldy-Willis, 1983.)

tightness and strength before coming to the conclusion that there is a problem with the sacroiliac joint. These muscles will be tested later under the examination of the hip joint.

THE HIP

The hip joint is the major ball-and-socket joint in the body. When compared to the shoulder, it is evident that the hip joint is built for stability and weight bearing, and the shoulder joint is designed primarily for mobility.

Bony Landmarks

The most significant bony landmark in the region of the hip joint is the greater trochanter and palpation of this structure is described below.

Greater Trochanter

This is the only palpable bony landmark associated with the hip joint. It can be palpated by running the fingers in a caudal direction from the waist on the lateral side. The greater trochanter is the first bony structure with which the fingers will come into contact. Its presence can be confirmed by asking the patient to medially and laterally rotate the hip at the same time as the therapist feels the movement beneath his or her fingertips.

Arthrokinematic Aspects of the Hip Joint

From the arthrokinematic viewpoint, the shoulder joint and hip joint are similar in that both the head of the humerus and the head of the femur are convex and, hence, will move in the opposite direction to the bone. Similarly, the glenoid cavity and the acetabulum are concave articular structures. The accessory movements occurring in the two joints are also similar. However, they are more difficult to achieve passively in the hip joint because of the size of the lower limb compared with the upper limb, and because the femoral head is deeply embedded in the acetabulum.

In the hip joint:

- an inferior glide of the femoral head accompanies flexion and abduction.
- a posterior glide facilitates flexion and medial rotation; an anterior glide facilitates extension and lateral rotation.
- lateral distraction facilitates all movements of the hip joint.

Two Important Angles Associated With the Hip Joint

1. *The angle of inclination.* This is the medial angle formed between the neck of the femur and the shaft. At birth, this angle is approximately 150°, but it reduces to 125° in the adult as a result of weight bearing. It has the effect of increasing the abductor lever arm, by moving the abductors away from the center of the hip joint, thus improving the efficiency of this muscle group. An increase in this angle (called coxa valga) will decrease the efficiency of the abductor muscles because they are brought closer to the center of the hip joint thus reducing the length of their lever arm. However, there is less stress on the femoral neck because the anatomical and mechanical axes lie in closer proximity. Conversely a decrease in the size of the angle of inclination (called coxa vara) has the effect of increasing the length of the lever arm and, consequently, the efficiency of the abductor mechanism. There is, however, more stress on the neck of the femur because the anatomical and mechanical axes are further apart.
2. *The angle of anteversion.* This is the angle created in the transverse plane between the head and neck of the femur and the shaft of the femur. It is easily observed by laying the femur flat on a table top and looking down along its length from the head down. It will be noted that the head and neck are angulated anteriorly compared with the femoral condyles and form an angle with a line drawn through the latter. This angle is the angle of anteversion, and it has an average range of 15-25° (Saudek, 1990). It has the effect of increasing the efficiency of the gluteus maximus muscle by increasing the length of its lever arm.

DETAILED EXAMINATION

Patient's Medical History

Although the hip joint receives input from L2 to S1, it is mainly derived from the L3 segment (Grieve, 1983) and so may refer pain to the L3 dermatome.

In addition to the usual questions that would be asked relating to location, onset, and behavior of the patient's pain, it is important to focus on the following:

- any childhood hip problems the patient may have had. The reason for this is that osteoarthritis of the hip is the most common affliction in the joint, and childhood hip problems can predispose the joint to this type of arthritis in adulthood.
- back problems are interrelated to the hip joint, and questions regarding previous back problems need to be addressed.
- repetitive strain activities involving one hip more than the other can also be responsible for hip problems, and information regarding these need to be elicited.
- the effect of the problem on functional activities must be determined. For example, can the patient put on a sock or stocking? Is the patient able to sit comfortably for any length of time? How far can the patient walk without pain? Is the patient able to climb stairs comfortably?

Observation

The focus is on gait when first observing the patient. Is there an antalgic limp? Is the patient lurching toward one side? Is there loss of hip extension? What is the position of the patient's lower extremity during the different phases of gait? Is there excessive motion of the pelvis?

The next focus of attention is the pelvic levels. If one ASIS is higher than the other, is there an accompanying adductor tightness; or is there an abductor tightness on the lower side? Is limb length inequality present? Is the distance between the greater trochanter and the ASIS the same on both sides?

Observation in the supine position should also focus on ensuring that the pelvis is lying square with the limbs (Adams & Hamblen, 1990).

Functional Tests

The order of testing and the type of test are the same as in previous chapters.

Passive Movements

These are difficult to perform in the hip joint because the therapist has to control the weight of the lower limb.

Patient in supine Hip flexion is tested with the knee bent so that the calf rests gently against the posterior thigh; note is taken of the end feel at the hip joint.

Abduction is tested in the scan examination but it is advisable to repeat it. When testing adduction the other lower extremity should be moved out of the way.

Medial and lateral rotation are tested with the hip and knee bent to 90°; the end feel is once again determined.

Straight leg raising is tested in the supine position. If the hip flexion is more painful and limited with the knee flexed, a severe lesion at the buttock — "the sign of the buttock" — must be suspected (Cyriax, 1982).

Resisted Isometric Contractions

Patient in supine Resisted hip flexion stresses psoas and less significantly the quadriceps.

Resisted hip adduction will detect a problem with the adductors.

Resisted knee extension would implicate the quadriceps mechanism if a painful response resulted.

Resisted abduction, medial and lateral rotation and extension, if painful, could be indicative of secondary manifestations of a bursitis (Cyriax, 1982), but a primary problem involving any member of the individual muscle groups cannot be ruled out.

Accessory Movements

The accessory movements (Kaltenborn, 1989; Wadsworth, 1988) are difficult to perform because of the muscle bulk and the weight of the lower extremity. However, the use of a belt will facilitate the testing of these movements where problems arise.

Inferior Glide (Figure 10-2)

- *Position of patient:* Supine, lying with the hip in 90° of flexion and the calf resting on the therapist's right shoulder.
- *Position of therapist:* Sitting, or standing, by the patient's right side.
- *Grips:* The hands are interlocked over the thigh (slightly anteromedially) and as close as possible to the hip joint.
- *Procedure:* The therapist leans back to achieve an inferior glide.

Lateral Distraction

- *Position of patient:* Supine, lying with the hip bent to 90° with the knee relaxed.
- *Position of therapist:* The therapist stands at the patient's right side.
- *Procedure:* A padded belt is placed around the medial side of the patient's thigh (a towel can be used to provide the padding) and around the therapist's hips. The therapist gently stabilizes the patient's knee from the lateral side at the same time as he or she leans back on the belt.

Posterior Glide (Figure 10-3)

- *Position of patient:* The patient is in the supine position with the hip bent to 90° in slight adduction and the knee in easy flexion.
- *Position of therapist:* Standing at the right side of the patient.
- *Grips:* Both hands interlock over the patient's right knee.
- *Procedure:* The therapist's body moves over his or her hands as the glide is performed.

Anterior glide (Figure 10-4)

- *Position of patient:* The patient is in the prone position with the right knee bent.
- *Position of the therapist:* The therapist stands on the right side of the hip being tested.
- *Proximal grip (mobilizing hand):* The therapist's right hand is placed over the posterior aspect of the hip joint.

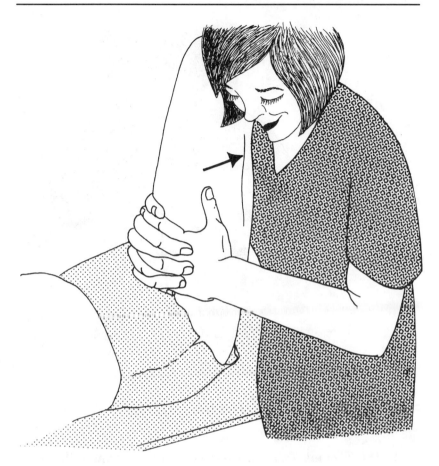

Figure 10-2. Inferior glide of the femoral head.

- *Distal grip:* This is a supporting grip. The therapist's left hand supports beneath the patient's right knee maintaining the right hip in neutral position.
- *Procedure:* The therapist moves his or her body weight over the right hand to achieve the anterior glide.

Special Tests

The following tests are commonly used when assessing the hip joint.

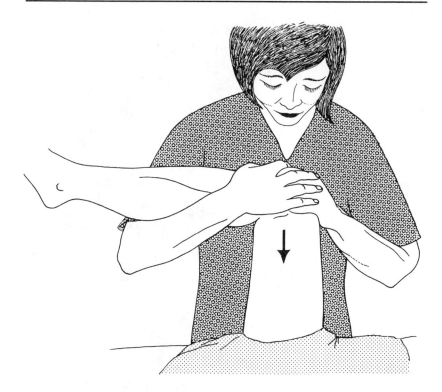

Figure 10-3. Posterior glide of the femoral head.

1. *The Thomas Test.* This test is used to determine the presence of tightness in the iliopsoas muscle.

- *Position of patient:* The patient is in the supine position with both knees held close to the chest.
- *Procedure:* The therapist instructs the patient to slowly extend the leg of the hip undergoing the test, as the other hip is maintained in flexion.
- *Result:* A positive result is obtained if the patient is unable to make contact between his or her posterior thigh and the plinth.

2. *The Rectus Femoris Test.* This is used to detect tightness in the rectus femoris muscle.

- *Position of patient:* The patient moves to the end of the plinth, in the supine position, and holds the left thigh in contact with the chest.

- *Procedure:* The patient tries to bend the right knee down as far as possible over the side of the plinth.
- *Result:* A positive result is obtained if the patient is unable to bend the knee, indicating tightness of rectus femoris.

3. *The Ober Test.* This test is used to elicit tightness in the iliotibial band. It is performed with the knee straight. If the knee is bent, the short fibers of tensor fasciae latae are under test.

- *Position of patient:* The patient is in the left side lying position with the knee extended.

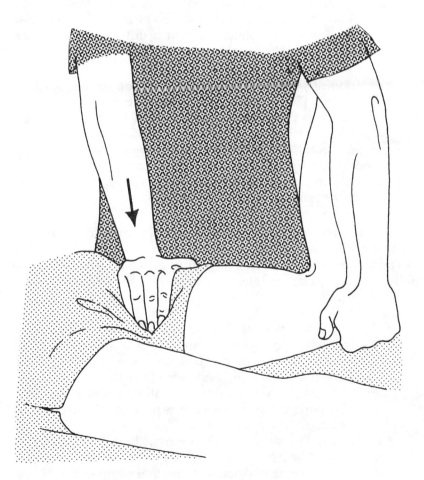

Figure 10-4. Anterior glide of the femoral head.

- *Position of therapist:* The therapist stands behind the patient.
- *Grips:* The proximal grip is over the upper pelvis to stabilize the hip. The distal grip supports under the medial side of the patient's leg.
- *Procedure:* The therapist extends the patient's right hip sufficiently for it to clear the under leg and allows it to fall into adduction with the knee straight.
- *Result:* If the patient's limb does not reach the plinth, there is tightness in the iliotibial band.

4. *The Fabere Test.* This is a combined movement of flexion, abduction, and external rotation. This test stresses the anteromedial capsule of the hip, but it also stresses the sacroiliac joint. If the patient complains of pain a differential test must be used to determine the exact cause.

- *Position of patient:* The patient is in the supine position.
- *Procedure:* The therapist passively places the heel of the hip under test on the anterior aspect of the patient's opposite thigh, such that the limb is in flexion, abduction, and external rotation.
- *Result:* Restriction of motion and pain would likely implicate the hip. If pain alone is experienced, the sacroiliac joint must also be tested.

5. *The Piriformis Test.* Of all the lateral rotators of the hip, piriformis seems to be the problematic member, probably because of its size and close proximity to the sciatic nerve. The following description relates to a procedure for tightness in the right piriformis.

- *Position of the patient:* Sitting on the plinth (or floor) with the left extremity extended and the hip and knee of the right limb flexed with the foot on the ground or plinth. The patient's left forearm extends along the lateral aspect of the thigh with the fingers pointing toward the right hip. The patient's right hand is resting on the ground behind the right hip (Saudek, 1990).
- *Procedure:* The patient pulls the right limb into medial rotation with the left forearm and hand.
- *Result:* If there is restriction of motion compared with the opposite side, tightness of the piriformis must be suspected.

Note: The above test has been chosen because the patient is able to use it, without help, to stretch the tight piriformis.

SUMMARY

In this chapter, the pertinent surface anatomy relating to the sacroiliac and hip joints was presented. Selected tests for common clinical asymmetries of the sacroiliac joint have been described. Passive physiological, resisted isometric and accessory movements of the hip, as well as special tests, were interpreted.

CHAPTER 11

The Knee Complex

The knee complex is composed of three different joints, the first two of which are integrally related in that both contribute to the intricate movements of the knee joint. The third joint does not contribute to the movements of the knee joint but is, nevertheless, intimately related to it. This knee complex consists of:

1. The patellofemoral joint
2. The tibiofemoral joint
3. The superior tibiofibular joint

First, several general aspects of the knee complex are discussed, such as surface anatomy, important points in eliciting a medical history, and observing the patient. The remainder of the chapter deals with specific aspects related to each of the three joints.

BONY LANDMARKS

The bony landmarks are easier to palpate if the patient is in the sitting position over the side of the treatment table. The therapist sits facing the patient.

Patella

The patella can be readily identified as an almost triangular structure with its apex pointing distally. A thick tendon descends from the patella; this is the infrapatellar tendon.

Anterior Portion of the Joint Line

If the therapist places a thumb in the depressions at either side of the infrapatellar tendon and presses inward, the anterior joint line can be palpated. This can be confirmed by asking the patient to straighten and bend the knee; movement will be felt at the joint line.

Tibial Plateaus

These plateaus are located just below the joint line and present as ridges. They are, in fact, the superior surface of the tibial condyles.

The Femoral Condyles

The condyles can be palpated by moving the thumbs upward from the joint line. It will be necessary to move medially a little to palpate the medial condyle and laterally a little to palpate the lateral condyle.

Tibial Tubercle

If the infrapatellar tendon is followed distally, a bony protuberance into which the tendon inserts can be palpated. This protuberance is the tibial tubercle.

Lateral Tubercle

This tubercle is located just below the lateral tibial plateau and lateral to the infrapatellar tendon. It is for the attachment of the iliotibial band.

Head of Fibula

If the therapist moves laterally from the tibial tubercle, the next bony prominence would be the head of the fibula.

PATIENT'S MEDICAL HISTORY

In addition to general questions regarding pain and onset (which are always asked when taking the history) the following questions need to be focused on, particularly if an injury was caused during an athletic activity (Clancy, 1985). The answers will give the therapist valuable information regarding the structure at fault.

1. "Can you remember which position your knee was in at the time of injury and what was the direction of the force?"
   - varus or valgus stress without rotation indicates collateral injury
   - twisting injury with a valgus or varus stress indicates possible meniscus tear with or without collateral injury
   - hyperextension injury indicates possible anterior cruciate injury
   - a fall on the flexed knee with the foot in plantar flexion indicates a possible posterior cruciate ligament injury.
2. "Did you hear any sound within the joint or feel something give?"
   - a "pop" is usually indicative of an anterior cruciate tear.
3. "Were you able to carry on with the activity?"
   - inability to do so indicates a serious injury (possibly an anterior cruciate tear).
4. "Did your knee swell? Soon after injury? Several hours after injury?"
   - swelling that occurs soon after an injury indicates bleeding into the joint and a serious injury, whereas swelling that occurs several hours later indicates effusion (synovial fluid) and a lesser injury.
5. "Does the knee lock?"
   - this suggests a meniscus tear.

6. "Does the knee give way?"
- this indicates instability due to injury of a meniscus or anterior cruciate or both.

OBSERVATION

The therapist should commence observation as the patient walks into examination room. Is the gait pattern normal? Is the patient favoring one leg more than the other?

Anterior Aspect

The therapist should look for the following signs. Is the patient exhibiting signs of genu varum (bow legs) or genu valgum (knock knee)? Are the patellae pointing forward or are they squinting? These observations indicate excessive medial rotation of the femur or excessive lateral rotation of the tibia; either will increase the Q angle (see p. 154-155) and, consequently, the lateral force on the patella. Is there obvious swelling about the knee? Is it local (extracapsular) or general (intracapsular)? Is the quadriceps bulk equal on both sides, or is there evidence of muscle wasting?

Lateral Aspect

The main observation to be made here is of the degree of extension of the knee. Is recurvatum present?

Posterior Aspect

Look for swelling in the popliteal space, which might reveal the presence of the synovial membrane piercing a weakened posterior capsule and forming a cyst-like structure. This condition is known as Baker's cyst. Sometimes, this is so large it extends down the back of the calf causing pain in that region.

DETECTION OF SLIGHT SYNOVIAL SWELLING

With the patient supine, first examine the knee joints in this position to note the presence or absence of the bilateral indentations at either side of the patella. Absence of these indentations indicates the presence of swelling.

1. The patient is supine with the knee relaxed in the extended position. The knee is stroked upward three or four times on the medial side commencing just below the joint line and extending upward to the suprapatellar pouch (this structure extends about a hand's width above the patella). Next, the lateral side of the knee is stroked downward from the suprapatellar pouch to just below the joint line. If present, fluid will pass to the medial side of the knee and bulge on the medial side of the patella.
2. Swelling in the suprapatellar pouch can be elicited by stroking several times over the pouch toward the knee and then compressing the pouch. If swelling is present, it will gather in the medial and/or lateral joint spaces.
3. To perform ballotement of the patella, the patella is tapped as pressure is maintained on the suprapatellar pouch. It will be felt to bounce in the presence of obvious swelling.

Normal Tracking of the Patella

Sit the patient over the side of the plinth, then do the following (Helfet, 1974).

1. Compare the normal tracking of the patella as the knee moves actively from the flexed position to the extended position. Note that it moves in a curve from a medial to lateral position to achieve its position on the trochlear fossa in full extension.
2. With the knee in the flexed position, put a mark on the middle of the patella with a skin pencil and one on the middle of the tibial tubercle (they should fall in a straight line). Ask the patient to extend the knee and notice how the mark on the tibial tubercle has moved laterally compared to the mark on the patella. Failure of the mark on the tibial tubercle to move laterally is indicative of loss of full extension.

THE PATELLOFEMORAL JOINT

This joint is formed from articulation between the trochlear surface of the femur and the posterior articulating surface of the patella. The patella is the largest sesamoid bone in the body.

Functions of the Patella

The four functions of the patella in the knee complex are:

1. To facilitate smooth movement of the tibiofemoral joint.
2. To improve the efficiency of the quadriceps mechanism by:
    a. "catching" the quadriceps as they move diagonally across the thigh and redirecting their line of pull along the longitudinal axis of the tibia.
    b. increasing the distance of the line of pull from the center of the joint thereby increasing the efficiency of the quadriceps.
3. To protect the anterior aspect of the tibiofemoral joint.
4. To provide a cosmetic effect to the tibiofemoral joint.

Biomechanics of the Patellofemoral Joint

The smooth movement of the patella is important in normal knee function. This movement is achieved by an intricate balance between the structures that surround the patella and are intimately associated with it. The quadriceps pull from above, and the pull of ligamentum patellae below create a vertical balance; the pull of the lateral forces (the retinaculum, the iliotibial band, and so on) are counteracted by the pull of the oblique and horizontal fibers of vastus medialis (Outerbridge & Dunlop, 1975).

The medial and lateral retinacula (fascial expansions from the quadriceps mechanism) maintain a medial and lateral pull on the patella. Tightness in either of these structures will exert a force on the patella in one direction or the other.

The Q angle (Figure 11-1) is the angle formed between a line drawn from the anterior superior iliac spine (ASIS) through the center of the patella and a line representing the upward extension of the long axis of the tibia, which also passes through the center of the patella. This angle creates a lateral force which is counteracted by the vastus medialis oblique (VMO). The fibers

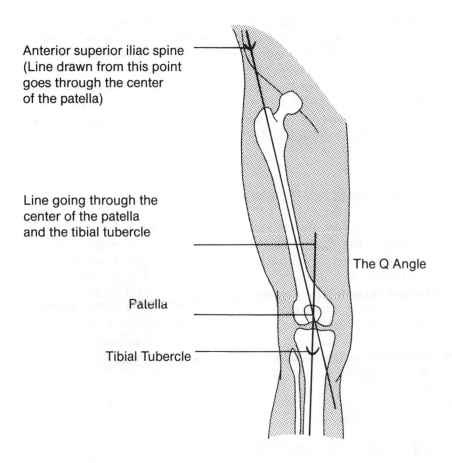

Anterior superior iliac spine
(Line drawn from this point
goes through the center
of the patella)

Line going through the
center of the patella
and the tibial tubercle

The Q Angle

Patella

Tibial Tubercle

Figure 11-1. The Q angle. (Adapted from Magee, 1987.)

of this muscle are inserted into the medial border of the patella
and extend about half way down this border. If the Q angle is
greater than 20°, there will be an increase in the lateral force.
Similarly, an abnormal insertion of the VMO (one that is
inserted too high on the medial border of the patella) will
decrease the effectiveness of the medial pull of this muscle. In
both instances, lateral subluxation or dislocation could result.

The ratio of the measurement of the length of the patella
and the ligamentum patellae should be approximately 1:1
(Kramer, 1986). If the length of the ligamentum patellae ex-
ceeds the length of the patella, a condition known as patella
alta (high riding patella) is present, predisposing the patella to

subluxation or dislocation. Conversely, if the ligamentum patellae is short compared with the length of the patella, a condition known as patella baja (low riding patella) exists, resulting in increased compression forces on the patella.

The enlarged lateral condyle of the femur helps to maintain the patella in a central position and prevents excessive lateral movement. However, if this condyle is underdeveloped, this lateral restraint is diminished.

Movements of the Patella

In full extension, the patella fits into the fossa on the trochlear surface of the femur. This surface extends downward onto the inferior surface of the medial condyle. When the knee is flexed, the patella is pulled down in such a way that it tilts away from the lateral condyle and the medial part of its articular surface rests against the medial condyle (Helfet, 1974). The smooth, downward displacement of the patella is important if full knee flexion of the knee joint is to be obtained. Similarly, since the movement of the patella is sinuous as it descends and ascends, medial and lateral movements are important.

DETAILED EXAMINATION

Accessory Movements

Distal Glide (Figure 11-2)

- *Purpose:* To test for restriction that would result in limitation of knee flexion.
- *Position of patient:* The patient is in the supine position.
- *Position of therapist:* The therapist stands at the side of the patient's knee with his or her back to the patient.
- *Grip:* The web between the index finger and the thumb of the left hand embraces the superior aspect of the patella. The therapist's right hand may be used to reinforce the left.
- *Procedure:* The therapist displaces the patella distally.

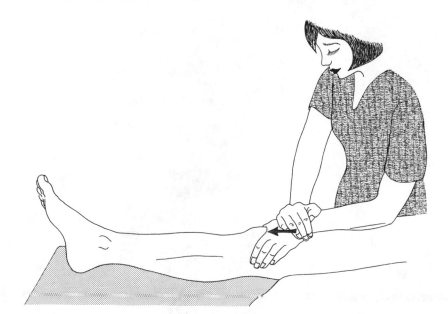

Figure 11-2. Distal glide of the patella.

Medial and Lateral Glides (Figure 11-3)

- *Purpose:* To maintain the mobility of the patella
- *Position of patient:* The patient is in the supine position.
- *Position of therapist:* The therapist stands facing the lateral aspect of the patient's knee.
- *Grips:* Both thumbs lie against the lateral border while the fingers lie in contact with the medial border of the patella.
- *Procedure:* The thumbs glide the patella medially while the fingers glide it laterally. Alternatively, the therapist can change sides and use the thumbs to glide the patella laterally. The lateral movement of the patella is also called the "Apprehension Test" because, in the presence of an unstable patella, the patient will show signs of alarm when this is performed.

Special Tests

The test described below is generally used to detect a symptomatic problem involving the articular surface of the patella.

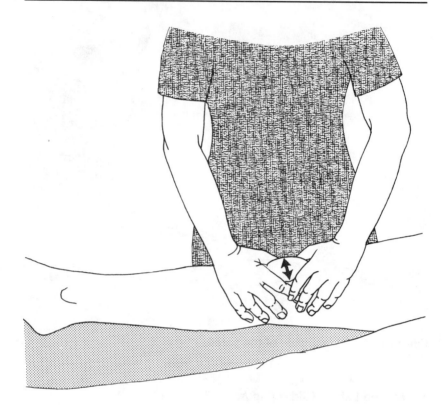

Figure 11-3. Medial and lateral glides of the patella.

Patella Compression Test (Clarke Test)

- *Purpose:* To test the integrity of the articular cartilage on the under surface of the patella.
- *Position of patient:* The patient is in the supine position with the knee in easy extension.
- *Position of therapist:* The therapist stands at the side of the patient at the level of the patient's knee.
- *Grip:* The therapist's left hand (web space between the index finger and thumb) embraces the proximal part of the patella.
- *Procedure:* The therapist gently displaces the patella in a distal direction at the same time as the patient is asked to contract the quadriceps. A painful response indicates problems on the articular surface of the patella (chondromalacia).

THE TIBIOFEMORAL JOINT

The tibiofemoral joint is formed by articulation of the femoral condyles with the tibial plateaus. The femoral condyles are separated posteriorly by the intercondylar notch; anteriorly, they blend to form the trochlear groove for articulation with the patella. In addition to flexion (accompanied by medial rotation of the tibia) and extension (accompanied by lateral rotation of the tibia), medial and lateral axial rotation can occur when the knee is in 90° of flexion.

Arthrokinematic Aspects of the Tibiofemoral Joint

The femoral condyles are convex and consequently move in the opposite direction to the movement of the tibia. The articulating surfaces of the tibia are concave and will move in the same direction as the bone. Deepening the tibial plateaus are the medial and lateral menisci; these are loosely attached to permit them to slide over the tibial surface.

The Menisci

General Features

Both menisci are semilunar in shape. The medial meniscus is described as forming a small part of a large circle; the lateral meniscus is said to form a large part of a small circle. The concave superior surfaces lie in contact with the femoral condyles; the inferior surfaces are flat and lie in contact with the tibial plateaus. The periphery of the menisci is spherical. As expected, the menisci are wedge shape in cross section.

Attachments From Anterior to Posterior

Both menisci are attached together anteriorly by the transverse ligament. The meniscopatellar ligaments extend from the patella to the menisci and are inserted into the latter anteriorly. The anterior horns of both menisci are inserted into the tibial plateaus. The anterior cruciate ligament sends fibers to attach to the anterior horn of the medial meniscus. The deep surface of the capsule inserts into both menisci. **The medial collateral ligament attaches to the medial meniscus but the lateral collateral ligament does not attach to the lateral meniscus.** Fibers from semimembranosis are inserted into the medial meniscus and fibers from the popliteus are inserted into the lateral meniscus. The posterior cruciate sends slips to the posterior horn of the lateral meniscus, forming the meniscofemoral ligament (Kapandji, 1987).

Movements of the Menisci

The menisci move forward during extension of the knee; they are pushed forward by the femoral condyles exposing the posterior part of the tibial condyles. Also, the meniscopatellar ligaments tighten during knee extension, and these ligaments will pull the menisci forward (Brownstein, Noyes, Mangine, & Sanford, 1988). During flexion of the knee, the menisci are pulled posteriorly; the medial meniscus is pulled by the semimembranosis; and the lateral meniscus is pulled posteriorly by the popliteus.

When the tibia rotates laterally on the femur during extension, the lateral femoral condyle moves forward on the lateral tibial condyle thereby moving the lateral meniscus forward; the medial femoral condyle moves posteriorly and so does the medial meniscus (Kapandji, 1987).

Functions

The functions of the menisci are:

1. to transmit the weight evenly through the knee joint.
2. to contribute to the stability of the knee joint (Fowler, 1976) by improving the congruence of the joint.
3. to act as shock absorbers.
4. to share the function of guiding rotation with the cruciate ligaments (Helfet, 1974) and, thus, to contribute to the movements of the knee.

DETAILED EXAMINATION

Since the history and observation of the knee complex have already been covered, the next stage in the detailed examination of the tibiofemoral joint is the checking of functional and special tests.

Functional Tests

In the acutely injured knee, the examination should be very gentle to avoid further damage to an injured structure (Keger-reis & Malone, 1988). In athletic injuries, the examination takes place on the field before swelling and spasm can develop. This is particularly so of joint stability tests (Andrish, 1985).

Passive Movements

Four passive movements are performed to detect problems with the inert structures of the tibiofemoral joint.

- Flexion
- Extension
- Medial rotation at 90° of flexion — excess range if the ACL is stretched or torn. Pain will be felt on the lateral joint line if the coronary ligament is damaged.
- Lateral rotation at 90° of flexion — excess range if medial collateral ligament is stretched or torn. Pain will be felt on the medial joint line if the coronary ligament is damaged.

Resisted Isometric Contractions

These contractions relate to the same movements as just listed and are best performed in the prone position with a pillow beneath the thigh to protect the patella. The knee is in 90° of flexion.

Accessory Movements

Traction

- *Purpose:* To test for hypomobility
- *Procedure:* The patient sits over the side of the plinth facing the therapist. The therapist grips the patient's leg with both hands just proximal to the malleoli and applies a sustained downward thrust to achieve distraction of the joint.

Posterior and Anterior Glides of the Tibia on the Femur These will be tested and compared during the "drawer tests" (see p. 164).

Medial and Lateral Glides of the Tibia on the Femur

- *Procedure:* The patient is in the supine position with the knee in about 25° of flexion. The leg is over the end of the plinth and the foot held between the therapist's legs. The distal femur is fixed by the therapist's proximal grip on the medial side. The therapist's distal grip is just distal to the joint line on the lateral side. The upper part of the tibia is moved medially with the femur fixed. The procedure is then repeated, with a change of hand position, to achieve a lateral glide of the tibia on the fixed femur (Kaltenborn, 1989).

Special Tests

Tests for Limitation of Physiological Extension

A slight limitation of extension is often difficult to detect; the following test is a useful one to perform with the patient in the prone position.

- *Procedure:* Ask the patient to move down the plinth so that the legs are extended over the end of the plinth, with the patellae free in space over the end of the plinth. The lower parts of the femurs are supported. In this position, the slightest loss of extension can easily be detected.

Ligamentous Stability Tests

Ligaments are divided into primary and secondary stabilizers for the different planes of knee motion (Brownstein et al. 1988). In the collateral stress tests to be described, the secondary restrainers for the medial collateral ligament are the posteromedial capsule (and associated structures), the anterior cruciate, and the posterior cruciate ligament. Those for the lateral collateral ligament are the posterolateral capsule (and associated structures), the anterior cruciate ligament, and the posterior cruciate ligament. It is, therefore, important to note the end feel during the performance of the tests. There will be an abrupt stop at the end of range if the primary stabilizer is intact. On the other hand, the end feel for a secondary stabilizer is soft and indistinct (Marshall & Baugher, 1980).

In some instances, more than one test is described for a particular ligamentous structure. This is because some therapists prefer one test to another, and all the tests described are seen in the clinical field. Where there are two tests for one structure, the advantages of one test over another will be discussed.

Collateral Ligament Stress Tests The tests used here are also known as the valgus and varus stress tests. In the former, an abduction force is applied to test the integrity of the medial collateral ligament. In the latter, an adduction force is applied to test the integrity of the lateral collateral ligament. The tests are performed initially with the knee in about 30° of flexion.

Medial Collateral Stress Test

- *Position of patient:* The patient is supine with the leg over the edge of the plinth.
- *Position of therapist:* The therapist faces the patient.
- *Proximal grip:* The therapist's left hand is placed on the lateral side of the lower part of the femur.
- *Distal grip:* The therapist's right hand is placed around the medial aspect of the lower tibia.
- *Procedure:* The therapist stabilizes the femur with the left hand at the same time as he or she applies an abduction (valgus) force with the right hand.

Note: In some instances the procedure can be facilitated by the therapist supporting the patient's foot between his or her arm and thorax, enabling the distal grip to be placed on the medial side of the leg. Movement of the therapist's body can then be used to apply the abduction stress to the tibia.

Lateral Collateral Stress Test

The position of the therapist's hands are changed so that the right hand supports the lower part of the medial femur and the left hand is placed on the lateral aspect of the lower fibula. An abduction (valgus) force is applied to stress the lateral collateral ligament.

Note: Excessive medial or lateral compartment opening indicates a torn medial or lateral ligament. The secondary restrainers are inactive, because they are slack with the knee in the flexed position. Next, the knee is extended (thus making the secondary restrainers taut), and the test is repeated. If the compartment opens in this position, there has been damage to the secondary restrainers also.

The Cruciate Ligament Drawer Tests The lateral profile of both knees in the flexed position (about 90°) should be observed to ensure the same starting position prior to testing.

Anterior Drawer Test

- *Procedure:* The patient is in the supine position with the knee flexed to 90°. The therapist sits on the patient's foot to stabilize it and to ensure that the hamstrings are relaxed. The upper part of the tibia is gripped with both hands, and the thumbs lie parallel to each other at either side of the ligamentum patellae. The therapist pulls firmly on the tibia and attempts a forward translation of the tibia on the femur. A positive result, indicating a torn anterior cruciate ligament, is obtained if a forward translation of the tibia occurs. O'Donoghue (1981) performs this test with the patient sitting over the side of the plinth with the patient's foot held firmly between his knees.

The anterior drawer test is unreliable in the presence of hemarthrosis or spasm of the hamstrings. Both will tend to prevent a forward translation of the tibia.

Brownstein and colleagues (1988) point out that during laxity tests, the amount of force used is much less than that normally acting on the knee, and even with the primary restraint gone only slight laxity may be evident on clinical testing.

Posterior Drawer Test (Figure 11-4)

- *Procedure:* The procedure is the same as that for the anterior drawer test, except the therapist attempts a backward translation of the tibia on the femur. A positive result is indicative of a torn posterior cruciate ligament.

The Lachmann Test for Anterior Cruciate (Andrish, 1985)

- *Procedure:* The leg is supported on a pillow in 15-20° of knee flexion and externally rotated to relax the hamstrings and the adductors. The lower end of the femur is stabilized with the therapist's proximal grip while the distal hand is placed beneath the upper part of the tibia,

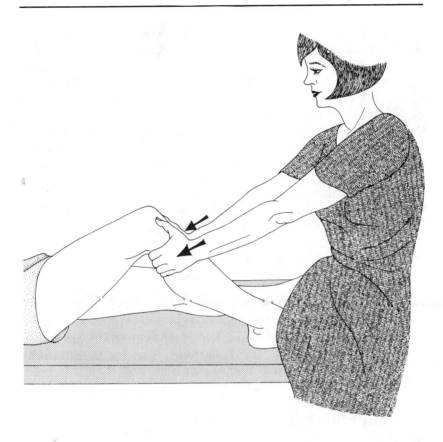

Figure 11-4. Posterior glide of the tibia on the femur.

to which an anterior force is applied. A forward translation of the tibia indicates that the anterior cruciate is torn.

The Lachmann test is considered more reliable because, in the position described, there is little opposition to the force exerted by the therapist and the results are, therefore, more credible.

Tests for Meniscus Injuries

The McMurray Test The McMurray test was originally developed as a test for the medial meniscus. It is currently used to test the integrity of the posterior part of either meniscus.

• *Procedure:* To test the posterior medial meniscus, the patient's knee is fully flexed with the patient in the supine position. The therapist's proximal grip is on the lateral aspect of the knee joint, with a finger placed on the medial joint line. The distal grip is above the ankle. The therapist laterally rotates the leg, applies a valgus force to the outer side of the knee and, maintaining the external rotation, slowly extends the knee. The sound of a click, or the feel of one on the medial joint line, indicates a posterior **medial** meniscus lesion.

To pick up a tear in the posterior **lateral** meniscus, the leg is internally rotated and a varus force is applied to the inside of the knee as the leg is extended.

The Apley Test   This test is preferred to the McMurray test by many therapists because it is considered more reliable.

• *Procedure:* The patient is in the prone lying position with the knee bent to 90°. The therapist applies a downward force to the sole of the patient's foot so that a compression force is applied to the knee joint. The leg is externally rotated to stress the medial meniscus and then internally rotated to stress the lateral meniscus.

THE SUPERIOR TIBIOFIBULAR JOINT

The superior tibiofibular joint tends to be ignored as a source of pain on the lateral side of the knee. Yet this joint and the distal tibiofibular joint provide the necessary rotation to enable the ankle mortise to decrease in size to accommodate the decreasing width of the posterior part of the talus during plantar flexion and the increase in size of the anterior part of the talus during dorsiflexion (Helfet, 1974). Similarly, the ankle mortise has to accommodate the movement of inversion and eversion of the foot, and this is again facilitated by movement at the tibiofibular joints.

Movements Occurring at the Superior Tibiofibular Joint

The compensatory motion that occurs at the superior tibiofibular joint to accommodate internal and external rotary movements of the tibia is threefold. There is a synchronous anterior-posterior movement, a superior-inferior movement, and a rotation of the tibia which is dependent on the position of the knee and the foot, that is, whether weight bearing or nonweight bearing.

These movements at the superior tibiofibular joint can be checked easily by sitting over the side of a plinth, with the thigh supported. Place your hand on the head of the fibula and note how it moves as you dorsiflex, plantarflex, evert, and invert the foot. (Radakovich & Malone, 1982).

DETAILED EXAMINATION

Accessory Movement

Anteroposterior Glide of the Head of the Fibula on the Tibia (Figure 11-5).

- *Position of patient:* The patient is in the left side lying position; the left extremity is extended, and there is relaxed flexion of the right hip and knee.
- *Position of therapist:* The therapist stands behind the patient at the level of the patient's knee.
- *Procedure:* The therapist supports the medial side of the patient's upper tibia with his or her right hand and the heel of the left hand lies against the posterior part of the head of the fibula. The pads of the fingers are placed in close proximity to the anterior aspect of the fibula.

  The heel of the therapist's hand moves the head of the fibula anteriorly and the pads of the fingers move it posteriorly.

Note: An alternative method is to have the patient in the supine position with the knee bent to 90° and the hip to 45°. The therapist sits on the patient's foot and stabilizes the knee by placing one hand on top of it as the other firmly grips the head of the fibula. The lateral side of the bent index finger is placed against the posterior aspect of the head of the fibula and the pad of the thumb against the anterior aspect of the head of the fibula. The fibula head is moved in a posterior direction from pressure of the thumb and moved anteriorly by the index finger. However, care must be taken with the peroneal nerve!

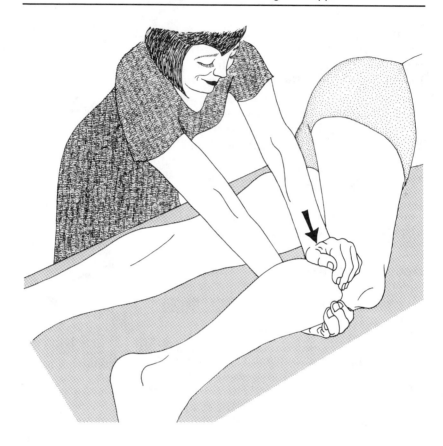

Figure 11-5. Anterior posterior glide of the head of the fibula on the tibia.

SUMMARY

In this chapter, pertinent anatomical landmarks were identified followed by specific information relating to the history of knee injuries. Focus then moved to observation of the joints in the complex and their detailed examination.

CHAPTER 12

Ankle and Foot Complex

ANKLE AND FOOT COMPLEX

The ankle and foot complex is composed of several joints; the most significant of these are the talocrural (ankle joint), the talocalcaneum (subtalar joint), and the midtarsal joint (talonavicular and calcaneocuboid joints). Injury commonly affects one or other of these joints and for this reason examination will be confined to them.

Bony Landmarks

For palpation of the bony landmarks the patient is in the half lying position and the therapist faces the sole of the patient's right foot.

Lateral Aspect

The therapist's right hand supports the medial side of the ankle and foot and the left hand locates the bony landmarks.

The Lateral Malleolus This is the bony projection located on the lateral aspect of the ankle. It embraces the lateral side of the talus and forms part of the ankle mortise.

The Sinus Tarsi This is a bony canal formed by the articulation of the talus and the calcaneum. It is located deep in a soft tissue depression lying just anterior to the lateral malleolus.

Neck of Talus If the foot is inverted, the neck of the talus can be located by palpating deep into the sinus tarsi.

Lateral Aspect of the Calcaneum This is the bony structure lying below the lateral malleolus.

Cuboid Just distal to the calcaneum, there is a depression. The cuboid bone can be palpated in this depression as can the calcaneo-cuboid articulation.

Styloid Process of the Fifth Metatarsal This can be located on the lateral aspect of the base of the fifth metatarsal just distal to the cuboid. It presents as a tuberosity, the purpose of which is to accommodate the insertion of peroneus brevis.

Medial Aspect

When palpating the structures on the medial side of the foot and ankle with the right hand, support is provided with the left hand.

Medial Malleolus On the medial side of the ankle joint, the medial malleolus can be found embracing the medial aspect of the talus. It does not extend as far distally as the lateral malleolus. Together, these two structures form the ankle mortise and embrace the talus.

Sustentaculum Tali This structure presents as a ridge about one centimeter below the medial malleolus.

Medial Aspect of the Neck of the Talus Distal to the medial malleolus, this structure can be palpated if the foot is placed in eversion.

Navicular Tubercle This can be felt distal to the neck of the talus on the medial aspect of the foot.

Medial Cuneiform The medial cuneiform articulates with the anterior aspect of the navicular proximally and distally with the first metatarsal to form the first tarsometatarsal joint.

The First Metatarsal This is easily palpated from the sole of the foot. The head can sometimes be seen as a bony protuberance on the dorsum of the foot, particularly in people with a high longtitudinal arch.

Arthrokinematics of the Ankle Joint and the Major Joints of the Foot

The movements of the articular surfaces of the following joints are in accordance with the concave convex rule.

The Ankle Joint (Talocrural Joint) Dorsiflexion of the foot is accompanied by a posterior glide of the talus, and plantarflexion is accompanied by an anterior glide.

The Subtalar Joint Supination, occurring at the subtalar joint, is accompanied by a medial glide of the anterior articular surface of the calcaneum (the anterior articular surface is concave). The posterior articular surface glides in a lateral direction, since this part of the articulation is convex.

Pronation is accompanied by a lateral glide of the anterior articulation on the calcaneum, because this part of the articular surface is concave. Conversely, the posterior articulation glides medially because it is convex.

The Talonavicular Joint The proximal articulating surface of the navicular is concave and that of the head of the talus is convex. It follows, then, that the navicular will move in the same direction as the physiological movement of the forefoot; the talus will move in the opposite direction.

During pronation, the navicular will glide in a plantar direction and laterally in an arc of movement; the talus will glide in a dorsal and medial direction. The reverse occurs during supination when the navicular glides in a dorsal and medial direction, and the talus glides in a plantar and lateral direction.

The Calcaneocuboid Joint This is a saddle joint in which the calcaneum is concave in a medial to lateral direction and convex in a dorsal to plantar direction.

The cuboid is convex in a medial to lateral direction and concave in a dorsal to plantar direction.

The talonavicular and the calcaneocuboid together form the transverse (or midtarsal) joint, which plays an important role in pronation and supination of the foot. In conjunction with the subtalar joint, the midtarsal joint assists the foot in accommodating to the different ground surfaces.

Close and Loose Packed Positions of the Ankle Joint

The close packed position for the ankle is dorsiflexion and the loose packed position is the neutral position. Hence, the foot is more stable when accommodated in a flat or low-heeled shoe than in a high-heeled shoe.

DETAILED EXAMINATION

The foot, like the hand, is a complex structure of joints and, as a result, is prone to numerous problems. Fortunately these problems can be revealed during assessment, and they usually respond to treatment.

Observation

It must be recognized at the onset that some of the manual tests utilized in the assessment of the foot and ankle may not reproduce the patient's problem. This is because the problem may only become apparent during weight bearing. It is, therefore, important that the during the process of observation, the foot and ankle be observed both in the weight-bearing and nonweight-bearing positions.

Weight Bearing

The patient's gait is observed for abnormal signs. Is there an antalgic gait? Is there interference with the normal performance in the sequence of events from heel strike to toe off? For example, is there normal extension of the great toe?

In the standing position, the foot is checked from behind, and note is taken of the position of the calcaneum and any deviation from the norm of the tendoachilles. If a line were drawn down the middle of the back of the calf and one down the middle of the tendoachilles, would they form a straight line? Is the heel inverting or everting? The longitudinal arch is observed for signs of pronation and the transverse arch for signs of depression. Note is taken of any abnormality relating to the toes, for example, hammer toes. Is the forefoot splayed?

Distribution of the body weight through the foot can be observed by asking the patient to walk where talcum powder has been sprinkled ("footprints in the sand"). Is the weight falling on the outer part of the heel and foot before crossing the forefoot to the head of the first metatarsal?

Ask the patient to go up on the toes, and note whether the heels invert. Ask the patient to assume the squatting position with the feet flat on the ground, and notice whether the foot goes into pronation. Next, get the patient to turn to the left in the standing position and note how the left foot will go into supination and that there is external rotation of the leg; the right foot goes into pronation, and this is accompanied by internal rotation of the leg. **It is a major function of the subtalar joint to convert the transverse rotations of the leg to either pronation (internal rotation) or supination (external rotation).**

The shoe should be examined, for example, the heel, the sole, the upper, the counter, and so on, for signs of inappropriate wear and poor design.

Nonweight Bearing

Attention is focused on the sole of the foot for signs of calluses and other problems, and on the dorsum of the foot for deformities of the toes.

Functional Tests

Passive Physiological Movements

During the performance of these movements the therapist takes note of the sensation imparted to her or his hand at the end of range.

The Ankle Joint (Talocrural Joint) Two passive movements are performed: ankle dorsi and plantar flexion. Passive ankle dorsi and plantar flexion will determine the range of motion. The end feel for both movements should be "soft," because of the antagonistic muscle tightness.

Talocalcaneal Joint The two movements tested at this joint are varus and valgus. The heel is cupped between the hands, and traction is applied to fix the talus in dorsiflexion (close packed position for the ankle joint) and eliminate movement at the ankle joint. The heel is turned inward to achieve the varus movement and outward to achieve the valgus movement.

Midtarsal Joint (Talonavicular and Calcaneocuboid Joints) The following four movements occur at this joint: dorsiflexion, plantarflexion, adduction, and abduction.

When testing the first two passively, the heel is cupped with one hand and pulled to fix the talus in dorsiflexion and prevent movement at the ankle joint. The mobilizing hand lies distal to the joint line.

When performing adduction and abduction, the talus and calcaneum are fixed with the proximal grip and the distal grip moves the navicular and the cuboid first in adduction then abduction.

Resisted Isometric Contractions

Resistance is applied to achieve isometric contractions of the dorsiflexors, plantarflexors, invertors, and evertors.

Accessory Movements

The accessory movements of the ankle joint are traction, dorsal and ventral glides of the tibia and fibula on the talus, and ventral and dorsal glides of talus in the ankle mortise.

The Ankle Joint

Traction (Figure 12-1)

- *Purpose:* To test for mobility through distraction of ankle joint
- *Position of patient:* The patient is supine with the foot in the resting position and extending over the edge of the plinth.

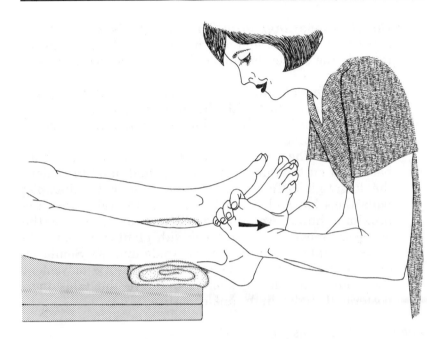

Figure 12-1. Traction of the ankle (talocrural) joint.

- *Position of therapist:* The therapist stands with one foot in front of the other, with knees bent, facing the sole of the patient's foot.
- *Grip:* The forearms are parallel, and both hands embrace the foot, one from the medial side and one from the lateral side, with the fingers overlapping on the dorsum of the foot. Thumbs are placed side by side on the sole of the foot lying parallel to the toes.
- *Procedure:* The therapist applies traction by pulling on the foot distally.

Dorsal and Ventral Glides of the Tibia and Fibula on the Talus

- *Purpose:* To test accessory movement and to increase plantar flexion (dorsal glide) and dorsiflexion (ventral glide) by mobilization.
- *Position of patient:* The patient is in the supine position with the knee bent and the foot in the resting position.
- *Position of therapist:* The therapist stands at the foot of the bed facing the sole of the patient's foot.

- *Distal (supporting) grip:* The therapist's thumb rests gently on the dorsum of the patient's foot pointing towards the ankle; the fingers lie in contact with the sole of the foot.
- *Proximal (mobilizing) grip:* The palm of the therapist's hand lies in contact with the lower part of the anterior aspect of the tibia with the fingers and thumb embracing the tibia and fibula.
- *Procedure:* The therapist moves the tibia and fibula backward on the talus with the proximal hand to achieve the dorsal glide. To achieve the ventral glide the therapist pulls the tibia and fibula forward on the talus with the proximal hand. An alternative way of assessing the accessory movement associated with plantar flexion is to move the talus anteriorly in the ankle mortise. Similarly, an alternative way to assess the accessory movement associated with dorsiflexion is to move the talus in a posterior direction in the ankle mortise.

Anterior Glide of Talus (Figure 12-2)

- *Position of patient:* The patient is in the prone position with the foot and ankle over the end of the plinth; there is a small supporting pad beneath the lower part of the leg.
- *Position of therapist:* The therapist stands on the lateral side of the patient's foot.
- *Proximal grip:* The web space between the index finger and thumb is placed just distal to the ankle mortise.
- *Distal grip:* The palm of the hand is placed on the dorsum of the foot, with the fingers lying around the medial border of the foot.
- *Procedure:* The therapist applies pressure with the proximal grip to achieve the anterior glide.

Dorsal (Posterior) Glide of Talus (Figure 12-3)

- *Purpose:* To test accessory movement.
- *Position of patient:* The patient is in the supine position, with the heel over the edge of the bed.
- *Position of therapist:* The therapist stands on the lateral side of the patient's foot.
- *Proximal grip:* The web space between the index finger and thumb lies over the talus, just distal to the ankle mortise.

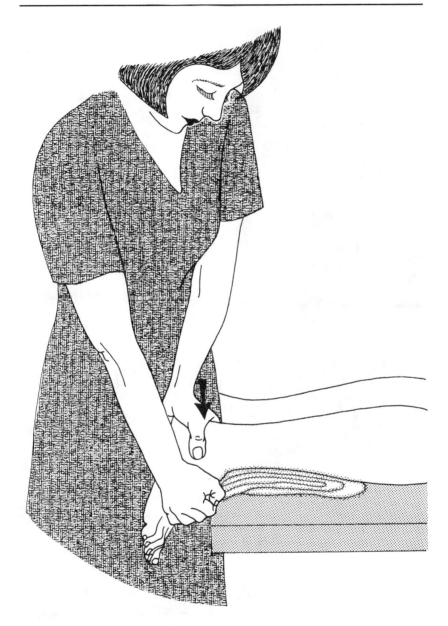

Figure 12-2. Anterior glide of the talus.

- *Distal grip:* The palm of the distal grip lies on the dorsal surface of the foot, with the fingers placed medially and the thumb directed laterally.

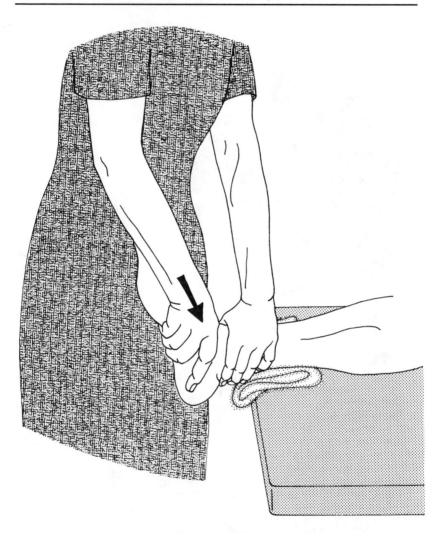

Figure 12-3. Posterior glide of the talus.

• *Procedure:* Slight traction is applied with the distal grip, as the hand glides the talus in a dorsal direction.

The Subtalar Joint (Talocalcaneal Joint)

Traction (Figure 12-4)

• *Position of patient:* The patient is in the supine position, with the heel over the edge of the plinth and the foot

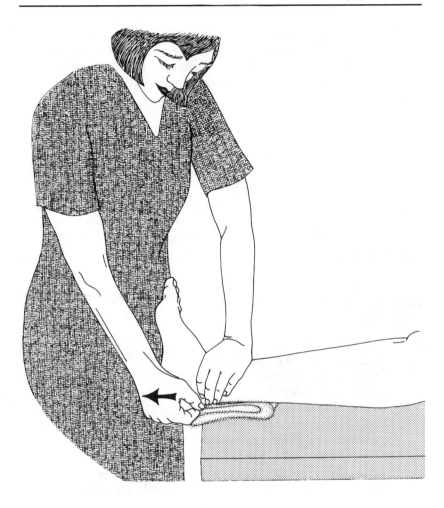

Figure 12-4. Traction to the subtalar joint.

supported in dorsiflexion by resting on the therapist's body.
- *Position of therapist:* The therapist faces the patient's foot.
- *Proximal grip:* This embraces the talus and the malleoli, holding them firmly.
- *Distal grip:* The distal grip is firmly around the calcaneum.
- *Procedure:* The therapist applies traction to the calcaneum in a direction which is parallel to the ground.

Medial and Lateral Glides of Calcaneum   It was pointed out earlier that the posterior facet on the calcaneum is convex, therefore, the posterior part of the calcaneum will glide laterally during inversion and medially during eversion.

Medial Glide (Figure 12-5)

- *Position of patient:* The patient is in the prone position, with a towel roll beneath the lower leg.
- *Position of therapist:* The therapist stands to the lateral side of the patient.
- *Grips:* The therapist's arms are in the outstretched position, the uppermost hand firmly grips the posterior calcaneum while the underneath hand embraces the anterior aspect of the ankle joint.
- *Procedure:* The therapist thrusts the posterior part of the calcaneum medially to facilitate eversion.

Lateral Glide

- *Position of patient:* The patient is in the prone position, with a towel roll beneath the lower leg.
- *Position of therapist:* The therapist moves to the medial side of the patient's foot.
- *Grips:* The therapist's arms are in the outstretched position. The uppermost hand firmly grips the posterior calcaneum while the underneath hand embraces the anterior aspect of the ankle joint.
- *Procedure:* The therapist glides the posterior part of the calcaneum in a lateral direction to facilitate inversion.

The Tarsometatarsal Joint

Dorsal and Plantar Glides

- *Purpose:* To test accessory movement and to mobilize
- *Position of patient:* The patient is in the half lying or supine position, with the foot in the resting position and the heel close to the end of the plinth
- *Position of therapist:* The therapist stands on the lateral side of the patient slightly proximal to the ankle.
- *Grips:* The proximal grip (therapist's left hand) fixes the cuneiform bones from the medial side with the thumb lying on the dorsal surface of the bones and fingers round the medial and plantar surface of the foot. The distal grip

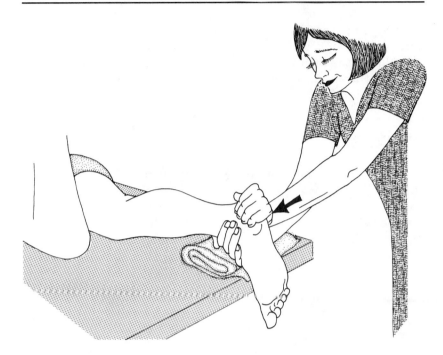

Figure 12-5. Medial glide of the calcaneum (posterior facet).

lies in close proximity with the proximal grip so that both thumbs and both index fingers are in contact. In this position the distal grip is in contact with the proximal part of the metatarsals.
- *Procedure:* The distal hand moves in a dorsal then plantar direction.

Special Tests

Ligaments

Medial Ligament   The deltoid, or medial, ligament is stressed by combined eversion and plantiflexion.

Lateral Ligament   The anterior lateral ligament (talofibular) fasciculus of the lateral ligament is stressed by combined plantarflexion and inversion.

The anterior drawer sign also tests for integrity of the lateral ligament. The patient lies supine with the foot clear of the plinth; the heel is gripped firmly by the therapist. The therapist's other hand fixes the tibia as he or she attempts to glide the talus anteriorly via the calcaneum.

SUMMARY

In this chapter, bony landmarks were identified on the lateral and medial aspects of the foot. This was followed by the arthrokinematics of the ankle and major joints of the foot. Next, the detailed examination was discussed including the importance of the weight-bearing position in the assessment process.

References

Adams, J.C., & Hamblen, D.L. (1990). *Outline of orthopaedics* (11th ed.). Edinburgh: Churchill Livingstone.

Andrish, J.T. (1985). Ligamentous injuries of the knee. *Orthopedic Clinics of North America, 16,* 273-284.

Backhouse, K.M., & Hutchings, R.T. (1986). *Color atlas of surface anatomy.* Baltimore: Williams and Wilkins.

Benjamin, A. (1969). *The helping interview.* Boston: Houghton Mifflin.

Bernstein L., Bernstein, R.S., & Dana, R. (1974). *Interviewing. A guide for health professionals.* New York: Appleton Century Crofts.

Bogduk, N., & Twomey, L.T. (1987). *Clinical anatomy of the lumbar spine* (2nd ed.). Edinburgh: Churchill Livingstone.

Bourdillon, J.F. (1982). *Spinal manipulation* (3rd ed.). London: Heinemann.

Brownstein, B., Noyes, R., Mangine, R.E., & Sanford, K. (1988). Anatomy and biomechanics. In R.E. Mangine (Ed.), Physical therapy of the knee. *Clinics in physical therapy. Volume 19* (pp. 1-3). New York: Churchill Livingstone.

Cailliet, R. (1988). *Soft tissue pain and disability* (2nd ed.). Philadelphia: F.A. Davis.

Clancy, W.G., Jr. (1985). Evaluation of acute knee injuries. In G. Finerman (Ed.), The knee. *American Academy of Orthopaedic Surgeons Symposium on sports medicine* (pp. 185-193). St. Louis, C.V. Mosby.

Cloward, R.B. (1959). Cervical diskography. A contribution to the etiology and mechanism of neck, shoulder and arm pain. *Annals of Surgery, 150,* 1052-1064.

Corrigan, B., & Maitland G.D. (1983). *Practical orthopedic medicine.* London: Butterworths.

Cyriax, J.H. (1982). *Textbook of orthopaedic medicine. Volume one. Diagnosis of soft tissue lesions* (8th ed.). London: Baillière Tindall.

Cyriax, J.H., & Cyriax, P. (1983). *Illustrated manual of orthopaedic medicine.* London: Butterworths.

Darnell, M.W. (1983). A proposed chronology of events for forward head posture. *The Journal of Craniomandibular Practice, 1*(4), 50-53.

Edwards, B.C. (1988). Combined movements of the cervical spine in examination and treatment. In R. Grant (Ed.), *Clinics in physical therapy. Volume 17* (pp. 125-151). New York: Churchill Livingstone.

Elvey, R.L. (1979). Brachial plexus tension tests and the pathoanatomical origin of arm pain. Aspects of manipulative therapy. *Proceedings of a Multidisciplinary International Conference on Manual Therapy, Melbourne, Australia.*

Fowler, P.J. (1976). Meniscal lesions in the adolescent. The role of arthroscopy in the management of adolescent knee problems. In J.C. Kennedy (Ed.), *The injured adolescent knee* (pp. 43-76). Baltimore: Williams and Wilkins.

Grant, R. (1988). Dizziness testing and manipulation of the cervical spine. In R. Grant, (Ed.), *Clinics in physical therapy. Volume 17* (pp. 111-124). New York: Churchill Livingstone.

Greenwood, P.E. (1989). *Principles of manual medicine.* Baltimore: Williams and Wilkins.

Grieve, G.P. (1981). *Common vertebral joint problems.* Edinburgh: Churchill Livingstone.

Grieve, G.P. (1983). The hip. *Physiotherapy, 69,* 196-204.

Hawkins, R.J., & Abrams, J.S. (1987). Impingement syndrome in the absence of rotator cuff tear. *Orthopedic Clinics of North America, 18,* 373-382.

Helfet, A. (1974). *Disorders of the knee.* Philadelphia: J.B. Lippincott.

Hoppenfeld, S. (1976). *Physical examination of the spine and extremities.* New York: Appleton Century Crofts.

Kaltenborn, F.M. (1989). *Manual mobilization of the extremity joints. Basic examination and treatment techniques* (4th ed.). Oslo: Olaf Norlis Bokhandel Universitetsgaten.

Kapandji, I.A. (1982). *The Physiology of the joints. Volume one. Upper limb* (5th ed.). Edinburgh: Churchill Livingstone.

Kapandji, I.A. (1974). *The Physiology of the joints. Volume three. The trunk and vertebral column* (2nd ed.). Edinburgh: Churchill Livingstone.

Kapandji, I.A. (1987). *The Physiology of the joints. Volume two. Lower limb* (5th ed.). Edinburgh: Churchill Livingstone.

Kaput, M. (1987). Anatomy and biomechanics of the shoulder. In R. Donatelli (Ed.), *Clinics in Physical Therapy. Volume 11* (pp. 1-16). New York: Churchill Livingstone.

Kegerreis, S., & Malone, T. (1988). The diagonal medial plica: An underestimated clinical entity. *Journal of Orthopedic and Sports Physical Therapy, 9,* 305-309.

Kenneally, M., Rubenach, H., & Elvey, R. (1988). The upper limb tension test: The S.L.R. test of the arm. In R. Grant (Ed.), *Clinics in Physical Therapy. Volume 17* (pp. 167-194). New York: Churchill Livingstone.

Kessel, L. (1982). *Clinical disorders of the shoulder.* Edinburgh: Churchill Livingstone.

Kirkaldy-Willis, W.H. (1983). *Managing low back pain.* New York: Churchill Livingstone.

Kisner, C., & Colby, L.A. (1990). *Therapeutic exercise. Foundations and techniques* (2nd ed.). Philadelphia: F.A. Davis.

Kramer, J. (1981). *Intervertebral disk diseases: Causes, diagnosis, treatment and prophylaxis.* Chicago and London: Year Book Medical Publishers; Verlag Stuttgart: Georg Thieme Publishers.

Kramer, P.G. (1986). Patella malalignment syndrome: Rationale to reduce excessive lateral pressure. *Journal of Orthopedic and Sports Physical Therapy, 8,* 301 309.

Lee, D. (1989). *The pelvic girdle.* Edinburgh: Churchill Livingstone.

MacConaill, M.A., & Basmajian, J.V. (1977). *Muscles and movements: A basis for human kinesiology.* Baltimore: Williams & Wilkins.

Magarey, M.E. (1988). Examination of the cervical and thoracic spine. In R. Grant (Ed.), *Clinics in physical therapy. Volume 17* (pp. 81-109). New York: Churchill Livingstone.

Magee, D.J. (1987). *Orthopedic physical assessment.* Philadelphia: W.B. Saunders.

Maigne, R. (1972). *Orthopedic medicine: A new approach to vertebral manipulation.* Springfield, IL: Charles C. Thomas.

Maitland, G.D. (1986). *Vertebral manipulation* (5th ed.). London: Butterworths.

Marshall, J.L., & Baugher, W.H. (1980). Stability examination of the knee: A simple anatomic approach. *Clinical Orthopaedics and Related Research, 146,* 78-83.

McKenzie, R.A. (1981). *The lumbar spine. Mechanical diagnosis and therapy.* Waikanae, New Zealand: Spinal Publications.

McKenzie, R.A. (1990). *The cervical and thoracic spine. Mechanical diagnosis and therapy.* Waikanae, New Zealand: Spinal Publications.

Mennell, J. McM. (1964). *Joint pain: Diagnosis and treatment using manipulation techniques.* Boston: Little, Brown.

Mitchell, F.L., Moran, P.S., & Pruzzo, N.A. (1979). *An evaluation and treatment manual of osteopathic muscle energy procedures.* Valley Park, Mitchell, Moran, and Pruzzo, Associates.

Neer, C.S., II. (1983). Impingement lesions. *Clinical Orthopaedics and Related Research, 173,* 70-77.

Neviaser, T.J. (1987). The role of the biceps tendon in the impingement syndrome. *Orthopedic Clinics of North America, 18,* 383-386.

Norkin, C., & Levangie, P. (1983). *Joint structure and function. A comprehensive analysis.* Philadelphia: F.A. Davis.

O'Donoghue, D.H. (1981). Diagnosis and treatment of injury to the anterior cruciate ligament. *Journal of Orthopaedic and Sports Physical Therapy, 1,* 100-105.

Outerbridge, R.E., & Dunlop, J.A.Y. (1975). The problem of chondromalacia patellae. *Clinical Orthopaedics and Related Research, 110,* 177-196.

Peat, M. (1986). Functional anatomy of the shoulder complex. *Physical Therapy, 66,* 1855- 1865.

Radakovich, M., & Malone, T. (1982). The superior tibiofibular joint: The forgotten joint. *Journal of Orthopedic and Sports Physical Therapy, 3,* 129-132.

Riordan, D.C. (1983). Functional anatomy of the hand and forearm. In J.S. Boswick, Jr., (Ed.), *Current concepts in hand surgery* (pp. 1-5). Philadelphia: Lea & Febiger.

Sarrafian, S.K., Melamed, J.L., & Goshgarian, G.M. (1977). Study of wrist motion in flexion and extension. *Clinical Orthopedics and Related Research, 126,* 153-159.

Saudek, C.E., (1990). The hip. In J.S. Gould III (Ed.), *Orthopaedic and sports physical therapy* (2nd ed., pp. 347-394). Philadelphia: C.V. Mosby.

Schwartz, E., Warren, R.F., O'Brien, S.J., & Fronek, J. (1987). Posterior shoulder instability. *The Orthopedic Clinics of North America, 18,* 409-420.

Steindler, A. (1955). *Kinesiology of the human body under normal and pathological conditions.* Springfield, IL: Charles C.Thomas.

Tullos, H.S., & Bryan, W.J. (1985). Functional anatomy of the elbow. In B. Zarins, J.R. Andrews, & W.G. Carson (Eds.), *Injuries to the throwing arm.* (pp. 191-200) Philadelphia: W.B. Saunders.

Urban, L.M. (1986). The straight-leg-raising test: A review. In G.P. Grieve, (Ed.), *Modern manual therapy of the vertebral column.* (pp. 567-575) Edinburgh: Churchill Livingstone.

Voltz, R.G., Lieb, M., & Benjamin, J. (1980). Biomechanics of the wrist. *Clinical Orthopedics and Related Research, 149,* 112-117.

Wadsworth, C.T. (1988). *Manual examination and treatment of the spine and extremities.* Baltimore: Williams and Wilkins.

Wells, P. (1982). Cervical dysfunction and shoulder problems. *Physiotherapy, 68,* 66-73.

Williams, P.L., & Warwick, R. (1980). Gray's anatomy (36th ed.). Edinburgh: Churchill Livingstone.

Yanda, V. (1988). Muscles and cervicogenic pain syndromes: In R. Grant (Ed.), *Clinics in physical therapy. Volume 17* (pp. 153-166). New York: Churchill Livingstone.

Index